TEEN DISORDERS

What Is Autism?

By Elisabeth Herschbach

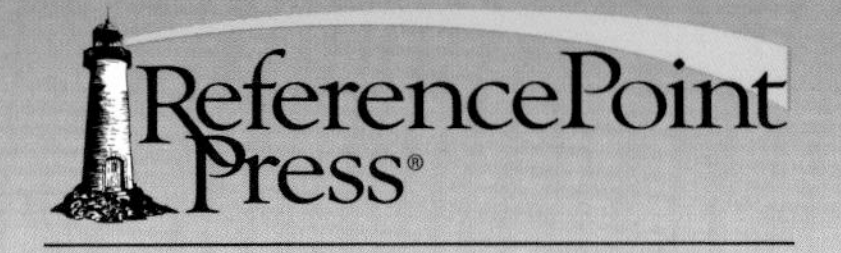

San Diego, CA

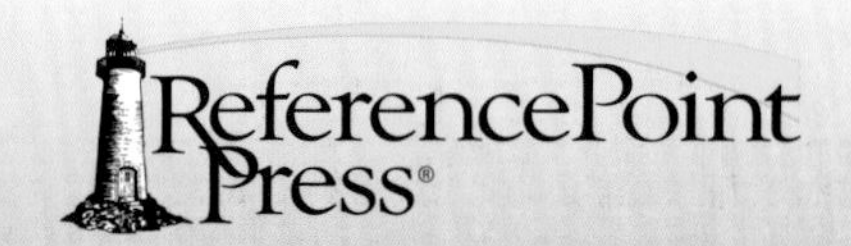

Printed in the United States

For more information, contact:
ReferencePoint Press, Inc.
PO Box 27779
San Diego, CA 92198
www.ReferencePointPress.com

Content Consultant: Bradley Ferguson, PhD, Assistant Research Professor, University of Missouri School of Health Professions

LIBRARY OF CONGRESS CATALOGING-IN-PUBLICATION DATA

Names: Herschbach, Elisabeth, author.
Title: What is autism? / Elisabeth Herschbach.
Description: San Diego, CA : ReferencePoint Press, [2021] | Series: Teen disorders | Includes bibliographical references and index. | Audience: Grades 10-12
Identifiers: LCCN 2020003543 (print) | LCCN 2020003544 (eBook) | ISBN 9781682829493 (hardcover) | ISBN 9781682829509 (eBook)
Subjects: LCSH: Autism--Juvenile literature. | Autism--Diagnosis--Juvenile literature. | Autism--Treatment--Juvenile literature.
Classification: LCC RC553.A88 H477 2021 (print) | LCC RC553.A88 (eBook) | DDC 616.85/882--dc23
LC record available at https://lccn.loc.gov/2020003543
LC eBook record available at https://lccn.loc.gov/2020003544

CONTENTS

INTRODUCTION

Struggling to Fit In

Growing up in Massachusetts in the 1950s, Temple Grandin was a creative, inventive child. She had a knack for art, and she loved designing and creating things. She spent hours alone building homemade kites, model airplanes, parachutes, and other ingenious contraptions out of makeshift materials. Once she even fashioned a helicopter out of broken bits of balsa wood. Its wind-up propeller launched it high into the air.

But while she excelled at such creative pursuits, Temple struggled with many aspects of daily life. Ordinary sounds and sensations were often overwhelming. They could even become painful for her. Certain types of clothing felt unbearable against her skin—"like sandpaper scraping away at raw nerve endings," as Temple later described it. Loud noises, such as the school bell ringing or balloons popping at a birthday party, were torture to her. The pain was "like a dentist's drill hitting a nerve," in her words.[1] Even minor background noise could be so distracting that she would find it difficult or impossible to concentrate.

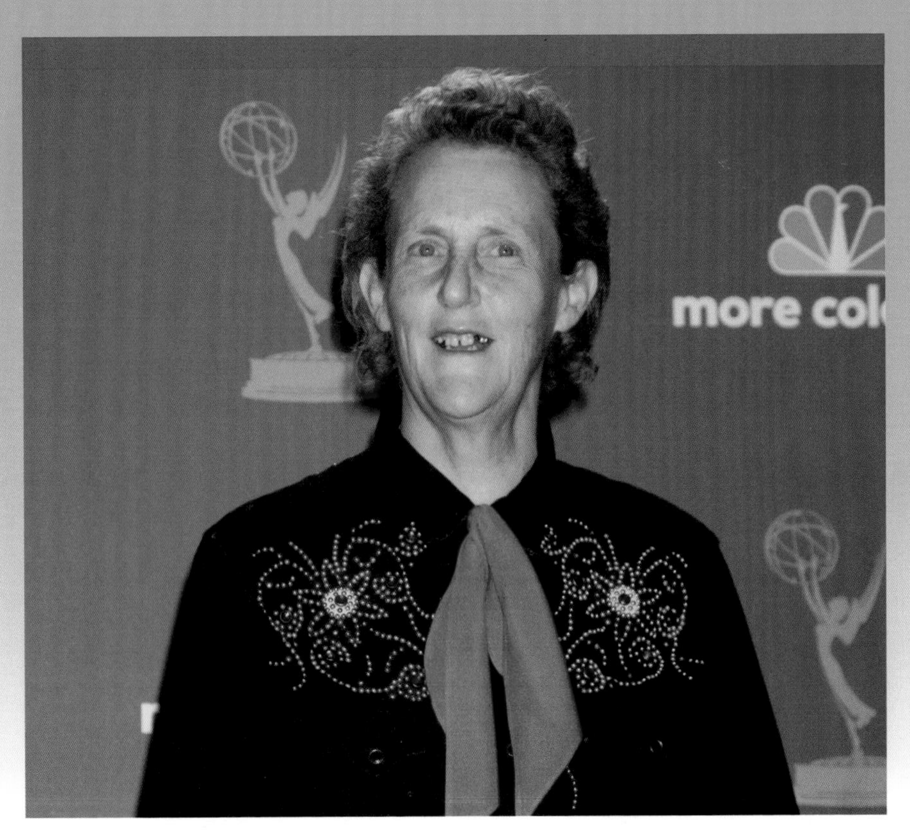

Temple Grandin is among the most publicly visible people with autism. She helped fight stigma by talking about the disorder.

Adjusting to junior high school was particularly difficult for Temple. Switching teachers and classrooms every hour was confusing and stressful for a girl who had trouble dealing with disruptions and changes in routine. Fitting in socially was even more difficult. Many of her classmates bullied her because of how she behaved. She spoke in a loud, flat voice and often repeated the same sentences and phrases over and over. She didn't look people in the eye and had trouble picking up on social cues. "I knew I did not fit in with my high school peers, and I was unable to figure out what I was doing wrong," she later wrote. "No matter how hard I tried, they made fun of me."[2]

> "I knew I did not fit in with my high school peers, and I was unable to figure out what I was doing wrong. No matter how hard I tried, they made fun of me."[2]
>
> *—Temple Grandin, professor and autism advocate*

These sensory and social problems were symptoms of Temple's autism, a developmental disorder that affects behavior, speech, and social interaction. From an early age, Temple had shown signs of being different. As an infant, she resisted being held, stiffening and recoiling when touched. She showed little interest in other people, instead staring off into space for extended periods of time. As a toddler, she threw violent tantrums, rocked, spun, and engaged in repetitive behaviors. She didn't speak until she was almost five years old.

Temple's father argued that they should put her in a psychiatric institution—a standard way of dealing with children like her in those days. Fortunately, however, her mother refused. Temple was given hours of speech therapy every week. An experienced nanny worked one-on-one with her to teach her basic social skills. By the time she was five, she was ready to attend a mainstream school. She went on to earn a doctoral degree in animal science.

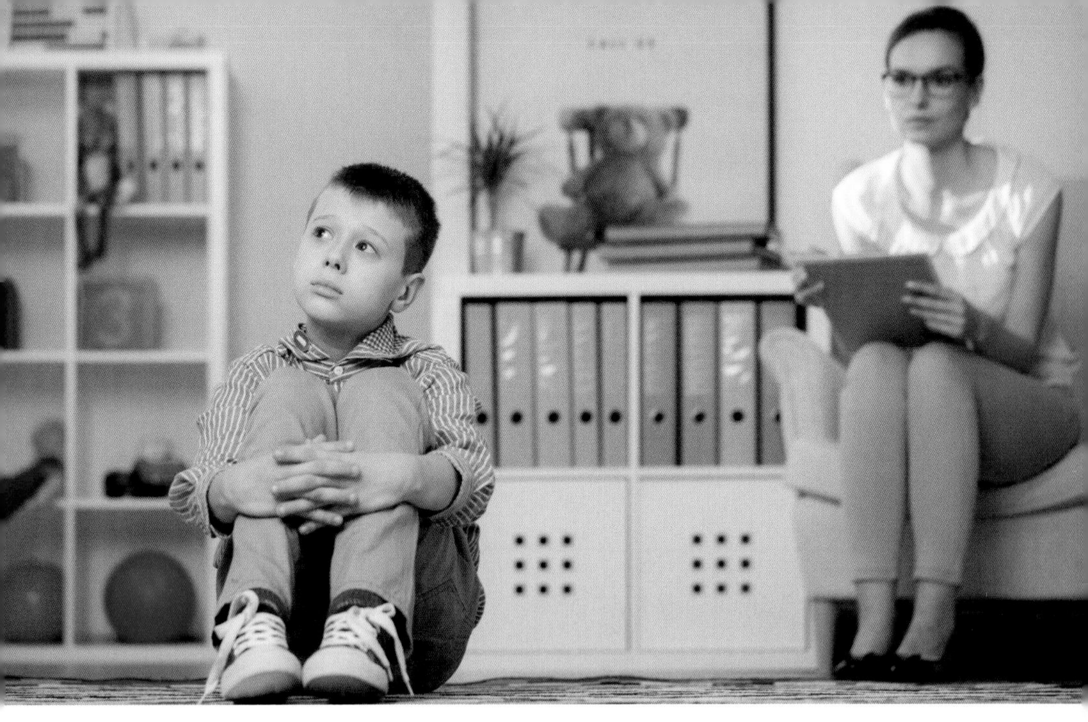

Kids with autism may have trouble interacting with others. However, Temple Grandin and other advocates have shown that these challenges should not limit what people with autism can hope to achieve.

Today, Temple Grandin is a distinguished professor at Colorado State University. She is a world expert in designing humane livestock-handling facilities, and half of all cattle-processing plants in the United States and Canada use systems she designed. She is also a world-renowned autism advocate. The author of several best-selling books, she flies around the world to give speeches and presentations on autism. By discussing her own experiences, Grandin has helped to change our understanding of autism and to lessen the stigma associated with it. "If I could snap my fingers and be non-autistic, I would not—because then I wouldn't be me," she says. "Autism is part of who I am."[3]

CHAPTER ONE

What Is Autism?

Little was known about autism when Temple Grandin was born in 1947. Just four years earlier, Austrian American psychiatrist Leo Kanner became the first to identify the condition as a distinct syndrome. In a 1943 article, the Johns Hopkins University psychiatrist described eleven young patients with unusual symptoms. The children showed "an inability to relate themselves in the ordinary way to people and situations," he wrote.[4] They seemed disengaged from their surroundings, absorbed in a world of their own. They moved in repetitive ways: banging their heads, spinning, rocking, flapping. Some of the children didn't speak. Others simply repeated certain words or phrases over and over. Because they appeared so withdrawn into themselves, Kanner described these children as "autistic"—from the Greek word *autos*, which means "self."[5]

Kanner introduced autism to the medical world. It took almost another four decades, however, for the condition to be officially recognized by mainstream psychiatry. In 1980, autism

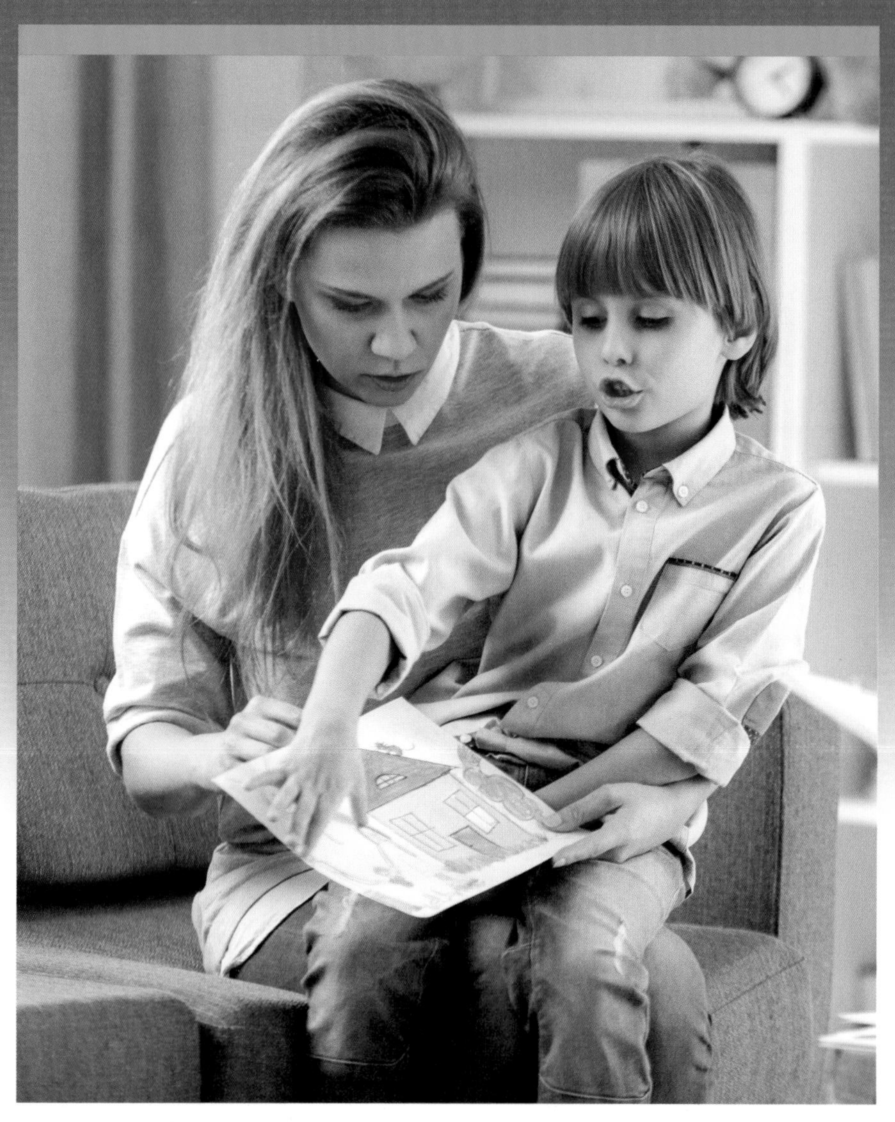

Leo Kanner identified autism in the 1940s. His ideas eventually developed into a recognized, diagnosable condition.

was included for the first time as its own diagnostic category in the *Diagnostic and Statistical Manual of Mental Disorders* (*DSM*)—considered the authoritative guide for diagnosing behavioral and mental disorders. Since then, the thinking about autism has continued to evolve. As research and clinical practice expand our understanding, health professionals continue to revise and redefine the standards for diagnosis in updated versions of the *DSM*. In 2020, the criteria used to diagnose autism were based on the fifth edition (*DSM-5*), published in 2013.

DEFINING AUTISM

Autism is considered a developmental disorder because it involves delays and impairments in typical developmental skills, beginning in early childhood. It is characterized as pervasive, meaning widespread, because it affects so many different behaviors and functions, with lifelong effects. And it is classified as a syndrome, as opposed to an illness, because it is defined in terms of a cluster of signs and symptoms rather than a single, specific underlying biological process.

The *DSM-5* groups these symptoms into two main areas. The first involves problems with social communication and interaction. These can take many different forms, ranging from impaired verbal and nonverbal communication skills to difficulties interpreting social contexts and relating to others. Like Kanner's young patients, autistic children may have trouble interacting with peers or family members. They may fail to make eye contact or to respond when addressed by name. They may struggle to interpret body language or other social cues. John Elder Robison, who was diagnosed with autism as an adult, describes spending hours memorizing facial expressions so that he could learn to replicate them. "I didn't even understand what looking someone in the eye meant," he writes in his autobiography, *Look Me in the Eye*. "And yet I felt ashamed, because people expected me to do it."[6]

> "I didn't even understand what looking someone in the eye meant. And yet I felt ashamed, because people expected me to do it."[6]
>
> —*John Elder Robison, who was diagnosed with autism as an adult, in his autobiography,* Look Me in the Eye

The second main area involves restricted, repetitive patterns of behavior, including ways of moving, speaking, thinking, and engaging with the world. For example, people with autism may have a tendency to rock back and forth, spin in circles, or flap their hands—repetitive motor movements commonly known as stimming. Children may interact with objects in unusual ways, such as lining up toys or flipping and spinning objects instead of engaging in more typical play. They may verbally repeat certain phrases over and over—a phenomenon known as echolalia. Many people with autism demonstrate rigid thinking patterns or inflexible adherence to routines, struggling with changes and transitions. Restricted interests are also common, such as the tendency to develop an intense, all-consuming interest in a narrow, very specific topic or activity.

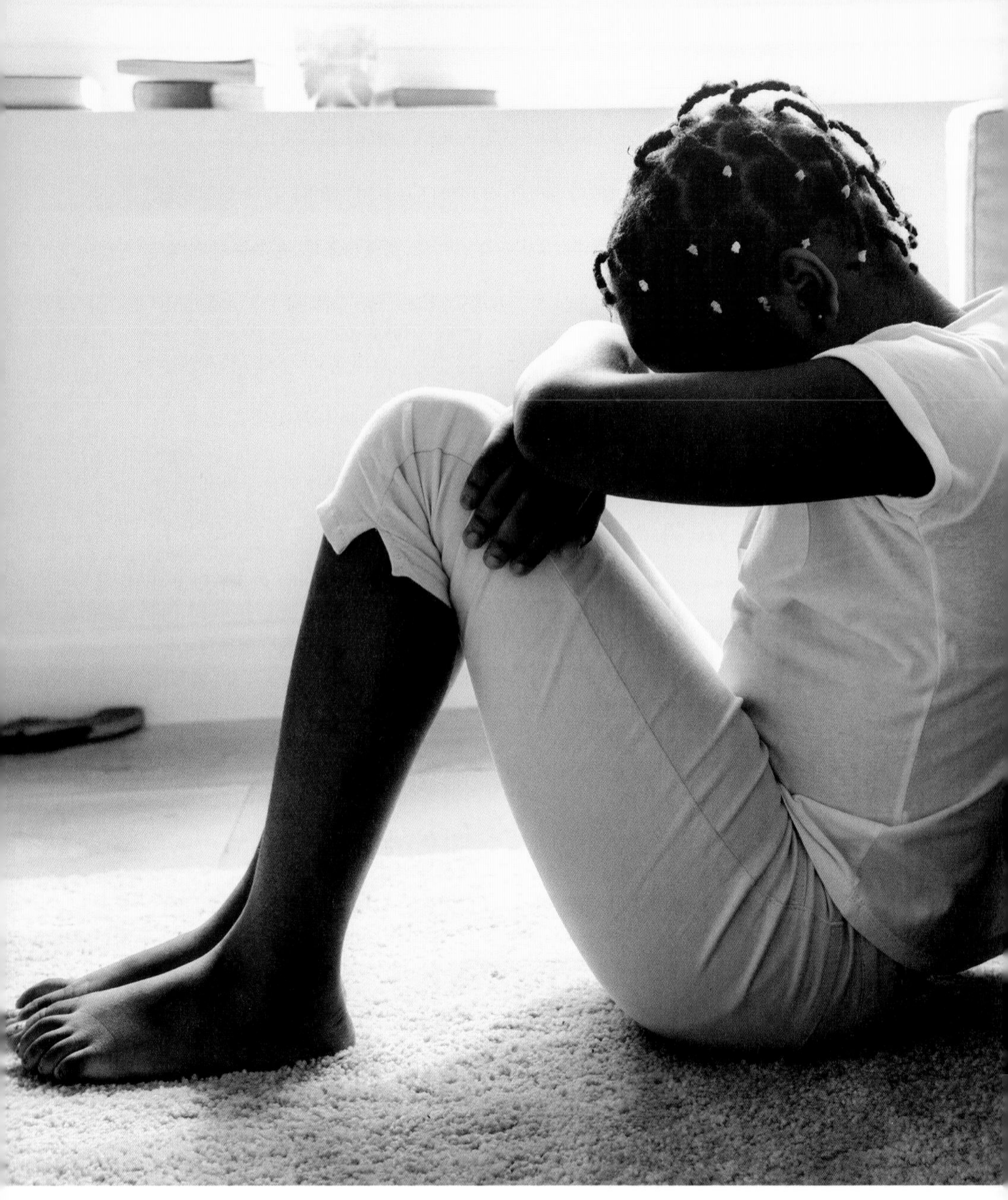

Those with autism may sometimes try to block out the outside world. They may feel overstimulated and overwhelmed.

Equally common are sensory processing problems, which the *DSM-5* also classifies under the category of restricted, repetitive patterns of behavior. For example, many people with autism are oversensitive to certain sounds, feelings, tastes, textures, smells, or visual sensations. In her first-person account of autism, *Thinking in Pictures*, Temple Grandin describes how her sensory problems intersected with other symptoms of autism during her childhood. Overwhelmed by too many environmental stimuli, sometimes she would break down into a temper tantrum. Other times, she would retreat into herself to block out the confusion of the world around her. "I would often space out and become hypnotized. I could sit for hours on the beach watching sand dribbling through my fingers," she writes. "I went into a trance which cut me off from the sights and sounds around me. Rocking and spinning were other ways to shut out the world when I became overloaded with too much noise."[7]

AN AUTISM EPIDEMIC?

When Temple Grandin was diagnosed with autism, the condition was considered very rare. Today, autism is considered one of the most common developmental disorders affecting children.

Current estimates of the prevalence of autism vary. According to the Centers for Disease Control and Prevention (CDC), one out of every fifty-nine children in the United States met the criteria for an autism diagnosis in 2018. The National Survey of Children's Health (NSCH) put the rate even higher, at one in forty children. That equates to some 1.5 million children nationwide.

Gender Gap

According to the CDC, boys are four times more likely to be diagnosed with autism than girls. In 2018, the CDC estimated that approximately 1 in 37 boys had autism. For girls, the rate was 1 in 151. Some researchers speculate that this may be tied to brain differences between males and females. But others think that many girls on the spectrum are simply getting missed. "The model that we have for a classic autism diagnosis has really turned out to be a male model," clinical neuropsychologist Susan F. Epstein says.[1] In girls, the symptoms can manifest somewhat differently. For example, girls tend to manifest fewer repetitive behaviors and a higher level of social engagement. Because they don't fit the stereotype, their symptoms can be mistaken for something else. Page, a mother to two autistic children, says that's what happened in her daughter's case. While her son was diagnosed at sixteen months, her daughter was not diagnosed until about five years of age. "We got a lot of different random little diagnoses," she recalls. "They kept saying, 'Oh, you have a girl. It's not autism.'"[2]

1. *Quoted in Beth Arky, "Why Many Autistic Girls Are Overlooked,"* Child Mind Institute, *n.d. www.childmind.org.*

2. *Quoted in Maia Szalavitz, "Autism—It's Different in Girls,"* Scientific American, *March 1, 2016. www.scientificamerican.com.*

Though the estimates differ, the consensus is that rates of autism diagnosis have risen sharply in the past few decades. In 1966, researchers estimated that roughly 1 in 2,500 American children had an autism diagnosis. By 2000, the prevalence rate had reached 1 in 150 children, according to the CDC. And by 2014, the estimate had more than doubled to a rate of 1 in 68. Between 2012 and 2014 alone, the CDC reported a 30 percent increase in prevalence. These numbers mirror trends around the globe, where rates of autism are estimated to have risen significantly worldwide since the 1990s.

AUTISM PREVALENCE

In 2018, the Autism and Developmental Disabilities Monitoring (ADDM) network released the results of a study on autism prevalence among eight-year-olds. It found higher rates of autism among boys compared to girls. Overall, it found that approximately one in fifty-nine children had been diagnosed with autism.

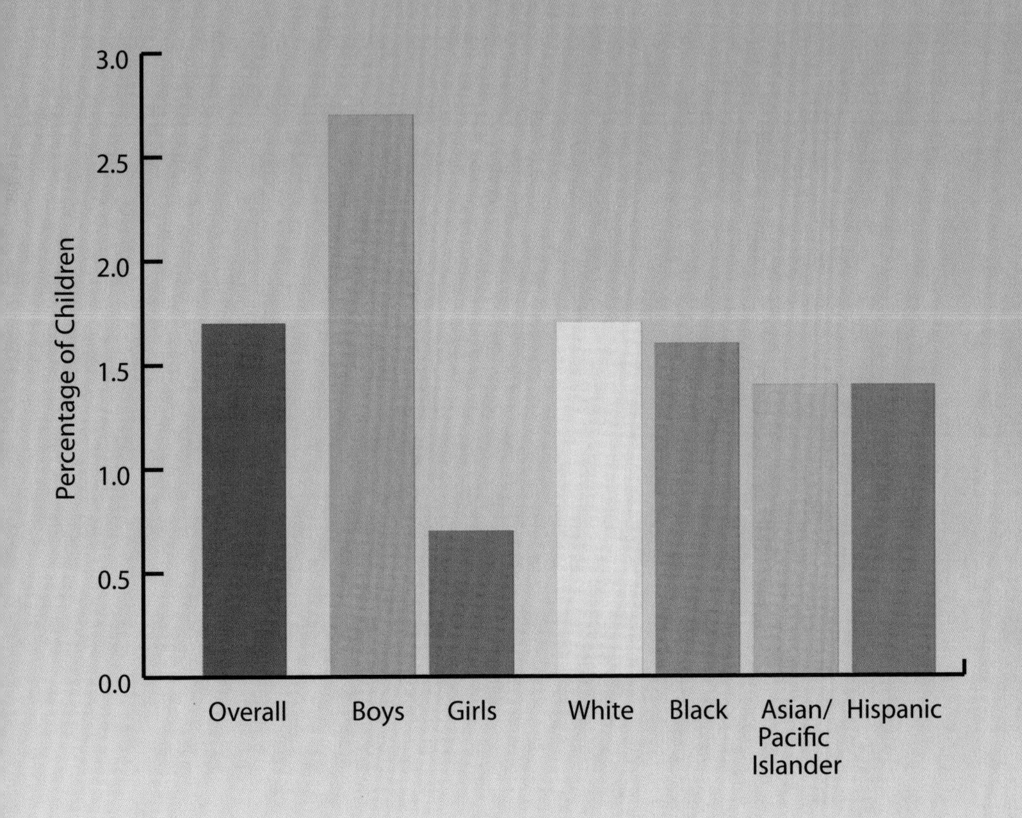

"Autism Spectrum Disorder," CDC, April 2018. nimh.nih.gov.

The spike in autism diagnoses has led some to warn of an epidemic. Many experts, however, think that much of the increase can be explained by other factors, including growing awareness and changes in the way the disorder is diagnosed. "There's greater awareness in the community around autism, more training of clinicians, more early childhood educators—that whole effort has increased awareness," says Coleen Boyle, director of the CDC's National Center on Birth Defects and Developmental Disabilities.[8]

> **"There's greater awareness in the community around autism, more training of clinicians, more early childhood educators—that whole effort has increased awareness."[8]**
>
> *—Coleen Boyle, director of the CDC's National Center on Birth Defects and Developmental Disabilities*

Increased awareness means fewer cases of autism are going undiagnosed as caregivers and doctors get better at identifying symptoms. At the same time, diagnostic standards have broadened. As a result, the autism label now applies to a wider range of cases. Some people now classified as autistic would have received other diagnoses in the past, including mental retardation. Some people with milder symptoms might simply have been regarded as odd or quirky. "Over the '80s and '90s, the diagnostic criteria expanded to include more children," says CDC researcher Daisy Christensen. "I think that's definitely a possibility for the increase that we've seen."[9]

A SPECTRUM OF SYMPTOMS

One reason that it is difficult to measure the prevalence of autism is that there is no definitive medical test for the condition. This makes it challenging to track and diagnose. Adding to the challenge is the sheer diversity of symptoms that can be involved. "We have no way to describe autism except by symptoms so variable that some clinicians refer to *the autisms*," writer Andrew Solomon notes.[10]

Both the specific symptoms and their severity can vary enormously from individual to individual. For this reason, autism is often referred to as autism spectrum disorder (ASD). The notion of a spectrum reflects the idea that symptoms fall along a continuum, ranging in degrees of severity. At one end of the autism spectrum, symptoms are so severe that they cause extreme lifelong disabilities, including nonverbal and self-injurious behavior. At the other end, symptoms such as difficulties in social situations may be so mild that they are hard to notice.

Although they are not official medical categories, the terms "high functioning" and "low functioning" are often used informally to describe the extremes of the spectrum. So-called high-functioning autistic people struggle with social interaction and have sensory issues and repetitive behaviors that may make them seem odd to others. However, they have typical or

Asperger's Syndrome

Milder forms of autism were once considered a separate diagnosis called Asperger's syndrome. Named after Austrian pediatrician Hans Asperger, Asperger's syndrome was added to the fourth edition of the *DSM*, published in 1994. The diagnosis applied to people who had difficulties with social interaction and communication but no language delay or cognitive impairments. In 2013, the *DSM-5* eliminated Asperger's syndrome as a separate category and merged it with the broader diagnosis of autism spectrum disorder. However, Asperger's is still included in the World Health Organization's International Classification of Diseases. And although it is no longer used for diagnostic purposes in the United States, the Asperger's label is still recognized in some countries elsewhere in the world. Recently, Swedish teen climate change activist Greta Thunberg has brought attention to Asperger's by publicly embracing her own diagnosis. "I have Asperger's and that means I'm sometimes a bit different from the norm. And—given the right circumstances—being different is a superpower," she stated.

Quoted in Allison Rourke, "Greta Thunberg Responds to Asperger's Critics: 'It's a Superpower,'" Guardian, *September 2, 2019. www.theguardian.com.*

even advanced language skills and no cognitive impairments. By contrast, people with so-called low-functioning autism are often unable to speak or are capable of only a few words. They have trouble learning basic skills, such as dressing themselves or taking care of their own hygiene. Even as adults, many need constant supervision and are incapable of living independently.

Autism symptoms can vary not just from one person to another but also in the same person over time. Like Grandin, some autistic children start out life with delayed speech and relatively severe symptoms but then go on to develop

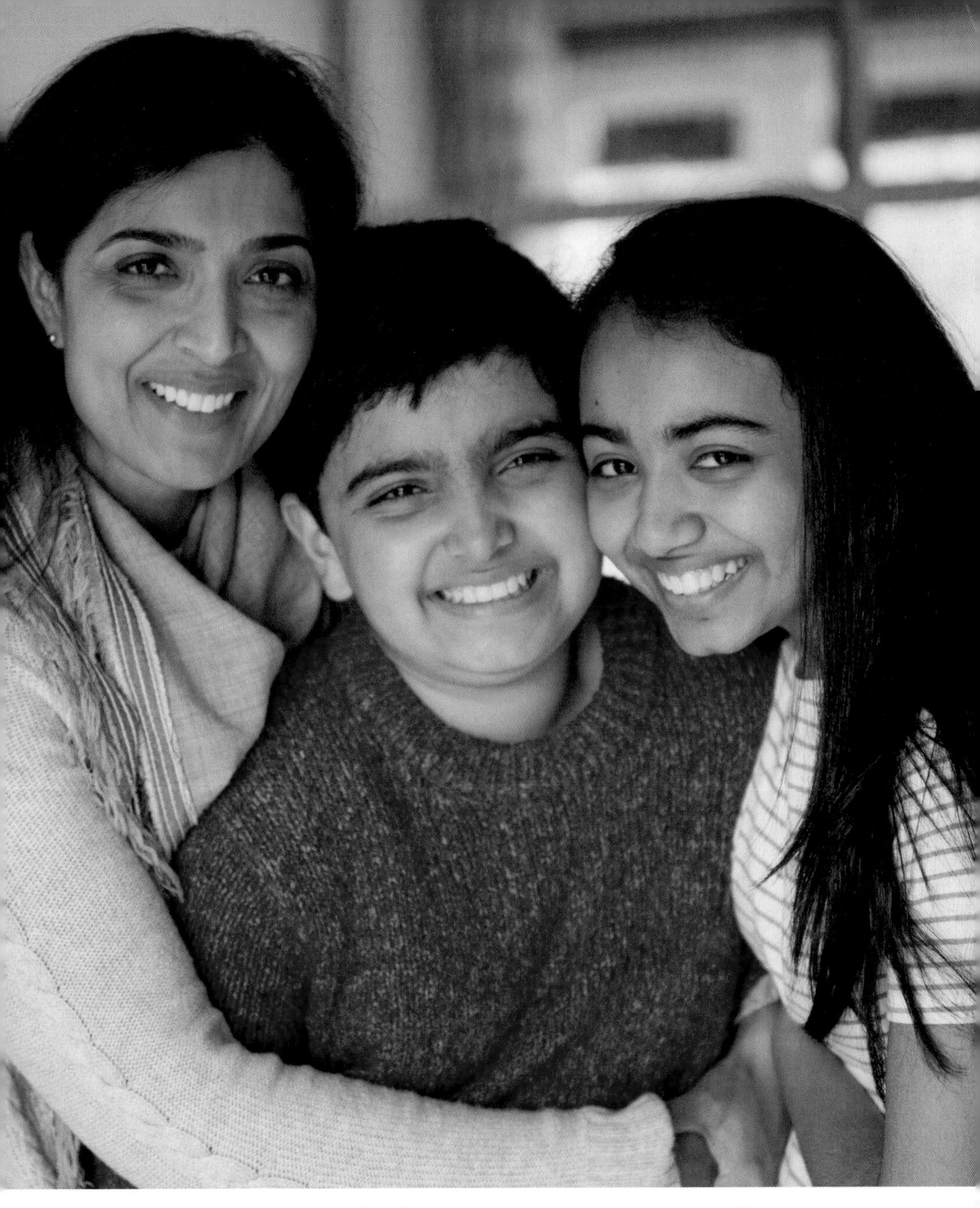

Autism symptoms can vary significantly from person to person. Different people may need very different levels of support in their daily lives.

normal language skills and become capable of a high degree of functioning. Researchers still don't understand exactly what determines the severity of symptoms—and why some people's symptoms improve with time and other people's do not. But one explanation for why some autistic people are unable to learn language is that their sensory processing problems are exceptionally severe. The sensory input they receive is so busy and distorted that their brains cannot accurately differentiate speech sounds.

It is thought that most people with nonverbal autism are intellectually disabled, with below-average mental functioning. Some individuals, however, may have average or even above-average intelligence but are unable to communicate their intelligence to others. In effect, they are trapped inside a sensory system that doesn't work. Ido Kedar, who cannot speak but learned to communicate with an iPad, describes the frustration of being presumed mentally deficient because of his inability to speak: "My intact thoughts don't transmit reliably to my motor system. I want to speak, but I cannot. This has robbed me of autonomy, imprisoning me within my own uncooperative body."[11]

An estimated one-third of people with autism are nonverbal, with no or only very limited speech. Some 30 percent of people on the autism spectrum are intellectually disabled, defined as having an IQ of 70 or below. About half score at or above an average level of IQ. Within these general ranges, however, there are countless shades of difference and degree along the continuum of autism symptoms. Every person on the autism spectrum has a unique constellation of behaviors, traits, and abilities. "It is regularly said that, when you have met one person with autism, you have met one person with autism," psychologist Lorna Selfe writes. "Every child diagnosed with ASD is at a different point along the spectrum and may be very different from another person with the same diagnosis."[12] This not only makes it difficult to define autism and to measure its prevalence, it also makes it challenging to identify the underlying causes.

"It is regularly said that, when you have met one person with autism, you have met one person with autism. Every child diagnosed with ASD is at a different point along the spectrum and may be very different from another person with the same diagnosis."[12]

—Psychologist Lorna Selfe

CHAPTER TWO

What Causes Autism?

For decades, doctors saw autism as a mental illness, a psychiatric disorder without any biological cause. Leo Kanner initially likened it to a childhood form of schizophrenia, a severe mental illness that causes hallucinations and delusions. Later, the prevailing theory among doctors was that so-called "refrigerator mothers" were to blame. According to this theory, popular into the 1970s, cold and emotionally distant mothers warped their children's development by failing to show them enough warmth and affection.

Today, the consensus among scientists is that autism is a neurological condition linked to changes in the developing brain that start before a child is even born. Researchers hypothesize that the core symptoms of autism stem from abnormalities in key areas of the brain responsible for regulating behavior, emotion, learning, memory, and cognitive flexibility. So far, however,

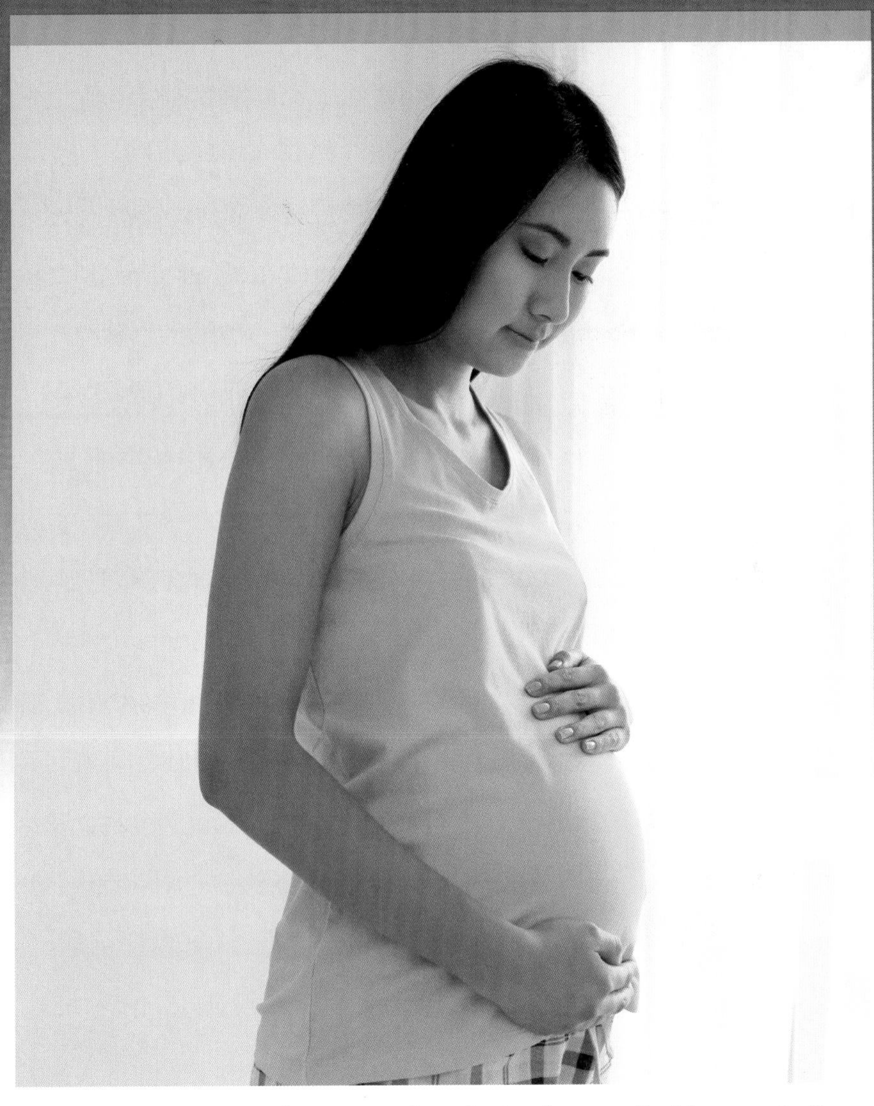

Experts believe that autism stems from brain changes that happen to the fetus in the womb. However, they are still studying what those specific changes might be.

no single theory has been able to fully explain the biological mechanisms that underpin this complex condition. “To this date, autism remains a diagnostic conundrum,” researchers Emily and Manuel Casanova state.[13]

THE NEUROSCIENCE OF AUTISM

The human brain is powered by roughly 100 billion neurons, specialized cells that communicate with each other along synapses, or pathways for sending and receiving electrical signals. Each of these billions of neurons communicates with thousands of other neurons at a time, using one of more than fifty different neurotransmitters. These are chemical substances that send signals from cell to cell, telling neurons how to respond. All these interconnected neurons are organized into dozens of structures that perform specialized functions, coordinating everything we think, feel, perceive, do, and remember. Each structure communicates with other brain structures, forming circuits, or loops of connected neurons, that shuttle information across different regions of the brain. The result is a vast network of constantly shifting neural connections far more complex than any computer.

> "To this date, autism remains a diagnostic conundrum."[13]
>
> *—Researchers Emily and Manuel Casanova*

This complexity is one reason it has been so difficult to map autism in the brain. Many different factors, from a person's environment and genes to their thoughts, actions, and experiences, shape the brain and its neural connections. As a result, even brains without disorders can vary a great deal. It can be hard to draw the line between normal variation and symptoms

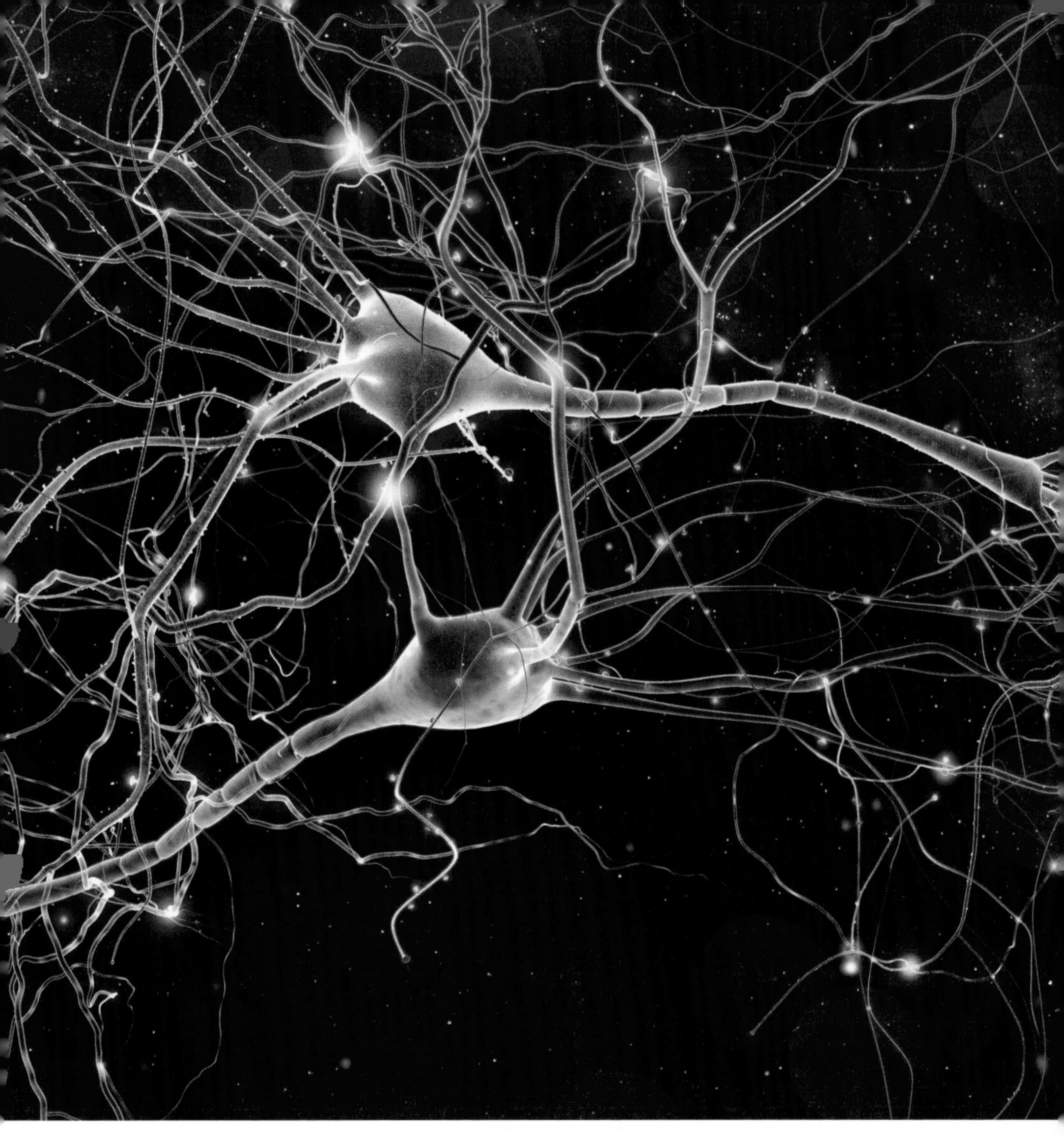

Researchers are studying the brain to discover what makes the brains of people with autism different. The connections between brain cells are particular areas of study.

of a disorder. And when differences are observed in the brains of autistic people, it can be difficult to tell whether these differences are caused by their autism or by something else.

As reported prevalence rates for autism rise, there has been a surge of research aimed at unraveling the causes behind

Mapping the Brain

Technological advances in neuroimaging give scientists increasingly sophisticated ways to see what's going on inside the brain. For example, functional magnetic resonance imaging (fMRI) enables researchers to measure neural activity in different areas of the brain. This helps them test how the brain processes information or responds to certain stimuli. Computed tomography (CT) scans take high-resolution pictures of the brain, allowing researchers to look for abnormalities in specific structures. High-definition fiber tracking (HDFT) reveals the detailed wiring of brain fibers, the bundles of nerve connections that link different areas of the brain.

Such technologies are putting an unprecedented trove of data into the hands of autism researchers. Interpreting the data is not always straightforward, however. For example, neuroimaging scans show that the temporal lobe, a part of the brain that specializes in facial recognition, differs in autistic people. Compared with nonautistic people, there is less neural activity in this part of the brain when autistic people look at faces. Do these weak neural connections explain the reduced social interaction characteristic of autism? Or does reduced social interaction—caused by some unknown factor—explain the weak neural connections? Brain scans by themselves can't tell us.

the disorder. Between 2008 and 2016 alone, funding for autism research increased 64 percent in the United States. Every year, scores of new studies add to a growing body of data pointing to subtle neurological differences that may be associated with autism. These include anatomical differences in specific brain structures as well as differences in the "wiring" of the brain—the patterns of neural connections that are formed.

Piecing all the data together into a consistent picture can be challenging. Different studies often report divergent—and sometimes contradictory—results. Thanks to advances in brain imaging technologies, however, some consistent patterns are starting to emerge. Several studies, for example, have identified abnormalities in the amygdala, an almond-shaped structure thought to regulate emotions, and in the cerebellum, a region that coordinates motor skills and visual processing, among other functions. Researchers have also identified structural differences in stacks of cells called minicolumns in the cerebral cortex, the hub for higher brain functions such as perception, attention, cognition, and language. The connected cells that form minicolumns are thought to be basic units of neural organization, similar to the microprocessors in computers.

MAKING CONNECTIONS

One of the most well-documented findings is an unusual enlargement of the brain in young children with autism. Most of this overgrowth appears to be in the prefrontal cortex, nicknamed the "command center" of the brain because of its role in thinking and decision-making. Studies have found that up to 20 percent of children with autism have significantly more neurons and synapses in this part of their brain during early development than their peers.

Some scientists hypothesize that these children start out with too many neural progenitor cells, or immature cells that are the precursors to neurons. These cells form while the fetus is still in the womb and then grow and divide into neurons as the brain develops. Another hypothesis is that something disrupts the brain's normal cycle of synaptic pruning—the process by which the brain prunes, or weeds out, unnecessary neural connections in order to work more efficiently. "You need to lose connections in order to develop a fine-tuned system of brain networks, because if all parts of the brain talk to all parts of the brain, all you get is noise," neuroscientist Ralph-Axel Müller explains.[14]

Either way, the surplus of neural connections is thought to interfere with normal social and cognitive development in young children. "You might think that having more synapses would make the brain work better, but that doesn't seem to be the case," says Azad Bonni, a neuroscience professor at Washington University School of Medicine in St. Louis. "An increased number of synapses creates miscommunication among neurons in the developing brain that correlates with impairments in learning, although we don't know how."[15]

While specific areas of the brain may be overconnected in those with autism, the two hemispheres of the brain appear to be underconnected. Research shows that children with autism have too many connections between nearby neurons, called local connections, but too few long-distance connections linking

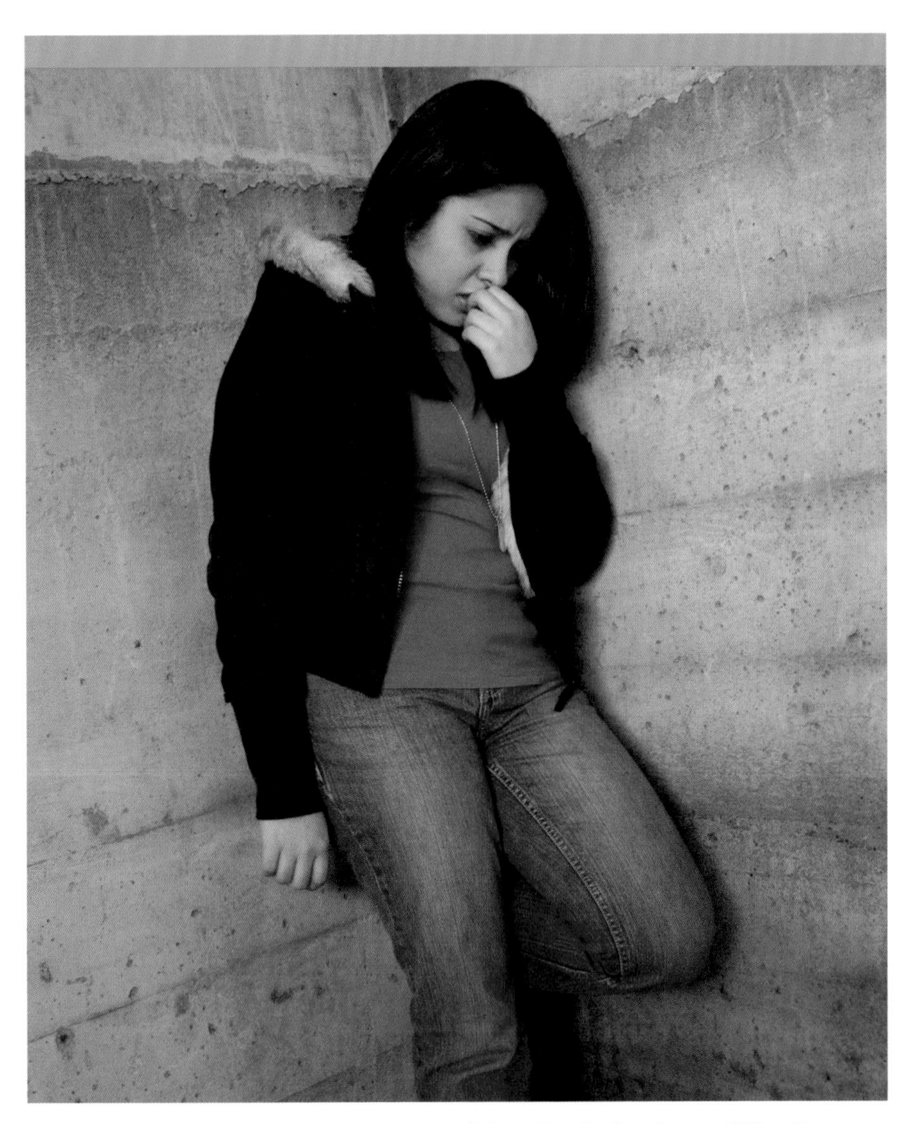

People with autism may be great at noticing details but have difficulty communicating with others. This combination can create problems with socialization.

distant areas of the brain. These long-distance connections are necessary for integrating information from different parts of the brain into a coherent whole. The result of this imbalance is that the brain becomes overloaded with a blitz of incoming information that it has trouble synthesizing, or putting together into a bigger picture.

"A preference for short-range connections over long ones emphasizes information generation. When this is at the expense of long-range connectivity, the brain isn't capable of integrating all the information it generates," the Casanovas explain in their book *Defining Autism*. "This may partly explain why autistic individuals are often attuned to details yet struggle with skills that require the coordinated efforts of multiple disparate brain regions, such as socialization, language, and motor movements."[16]

This theory fits with how many people on the spectrum describe their own subjective experience. "The challenge for autistic individuals is that they are overwhelmed even by their own minds. Typically they notice more details than other people," Kamran Nazeer writes in his memoir about living with autism. "Simultaneously, the ability of autistic individuals to categorize or process this information is more limited. . . . With this combination of high input and low output, inevitably a sort of logjam occurs."[17]

DIAGNOSING AUTISM

Autism researchers hope that identifying specific neural processes and brain structures that are involved in autism will

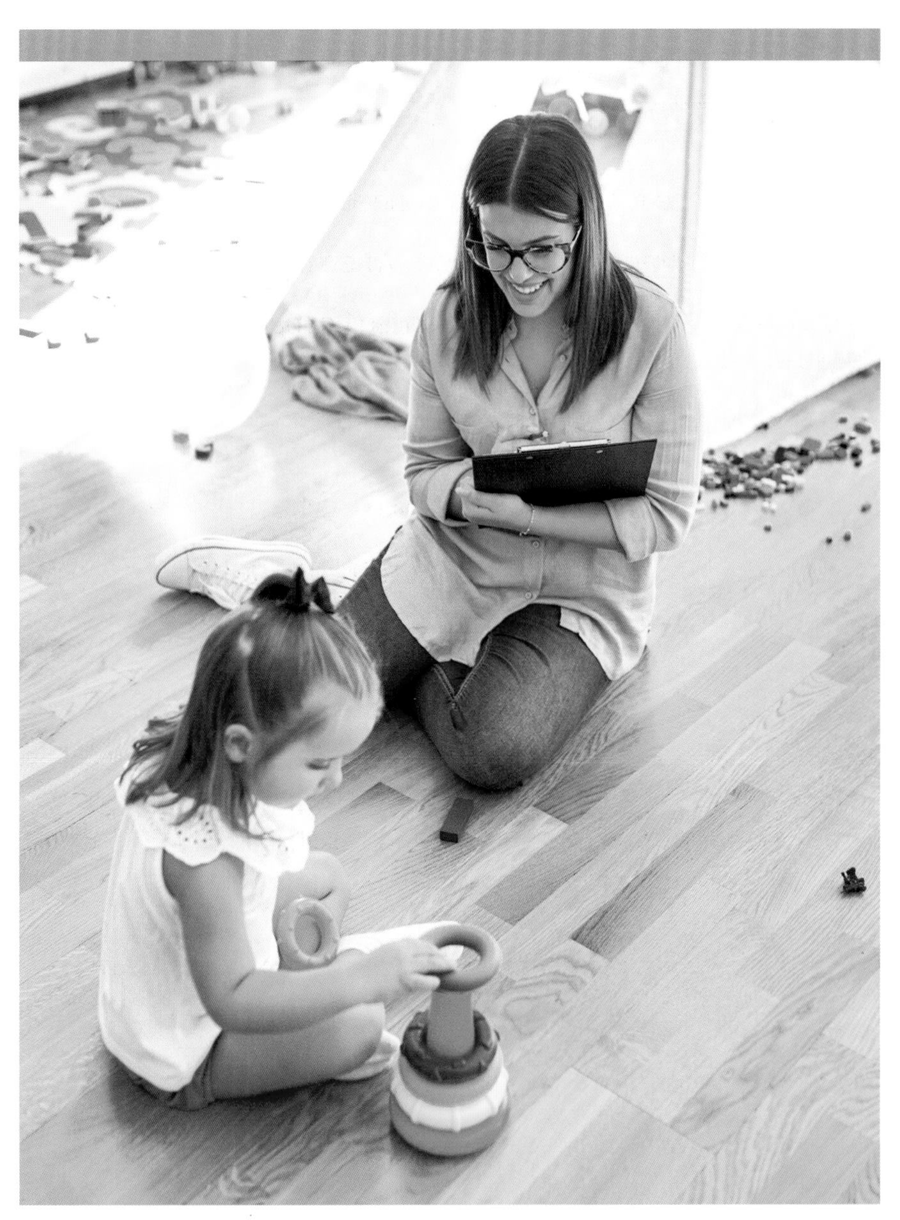

Psychologists observe children to diagnose autism. They use the criteria from the *DSM* in the diagnostic process.

lead to new ways of diagnosing the condition. Currently, doctors rely on behavioral screenings for diagnosis. Using a checklist or questionnaire based on the clinical standards established by the *DSM*, a team of experts will observe a child's behavior and interview his or her parents. The goal is to look for signs of developmental delays, deficits in communication and social engagement, and evidence of repetitive behaviors. Inevitably, there is an element of subjectivity involved in the process. And because it takes time for delays to become apparent and certain behaviors to emerge, it can be hard to diagnose autism before a child is eighteen to twenty-four months old. Most autistic children in the United States, in fact, are not diagnosed until they are over four years old.

Mapping out the neural pathways of autism would give doctors a way to diagnose the condition with an objective medical test that could detect signs of autism in the brain before any behavioral symptoms become apparent. Earlier detection would then allow for earlier treatment, which experts agree leads to the best outcomes.

Some promising avenues have already emerged. For example, researchers at King's College London used brain scans to measure the thickness of the cortex in test participants and were able to identify those with autism with accuracy rates of up to 90 percent. Another study showed that the volume of a certain type of spinal fluid was able to predict an autism diagnosis with an accuracy of about 70 percent. And a

Boston Children's Hospital research team has shown that autistic children have distinctive brain wave patterns that can be detected with an electroencephalogram (EEG), a simple, inexpensive test that measures electrical activity in the brain. By analyzing these brain wave patterns, doctors may be able to predict autism in children as young as three months old. "The results were stunning," lead researcher William Bosl says. "Our predictive accuracy by 9 months of age was nearly 100 percent."[18]

Despite such progress, however, doctors are a long way off from having any biomarkers—objectively measurable biological signs—for autism. "To diagnose autism reliably, we need to better understand what goes awry in people with the disorder," says Nicholas Lange, a Harvard Medical School biostatistician. "Until its solid biological basis is found, any attempt to use brain imaging to diagnose autism will be futile."[19]

"To diagnose autism reliably, we need to better understand what goes awry in people with the disorder. Until its solid biological basis is found, any attempt to use brain imaging to diagnose autism will be futile."[19]

—Biostatistician Nicholas Lange, Harvard Medical School

A persistent obstacle autism researchers face is that no single set of variables can explain all or even most autism cases. Not everyone with the same symptoms shows the same neurological features. And not everyone with the same neurological features manifests the same symptoms. "Even when researchers do think they've found a match between an autistic person's behavior and an anomaly in the brain, they can't be sure that someone else manifesting the same behavior would have the same anomaly," Temple Grandin writes in her book *The Autistic Brain*. "Conversely, when researchers find an anomaly in the brain, they can't be sure that that anomaly will have the same behavioral effect in a different brain."[20]

Most researchers now think there is no single underlying neurological basis for autism. Instead, autism is probably a collection of different disorders that produce similar behaviors but arise from different mechanisms in the brain. In turn, these brain mechanisms are caused by complex interactions between multiple factors, including both genes and the environment. As psychologist Christian Jarrett puts it, "the simple term 'autism' conceals a world of complexity."[21]

ALL IN THE FAMILY

Genes are strings of DNA, the basic hereditary material found in every cell. There are roughly 20,000 genes in almost every cell in the human body. Passed on from parents to children, genes act like a blueprint or set of instructions that tells the body how to grow and function. Scientists know that genes shape how

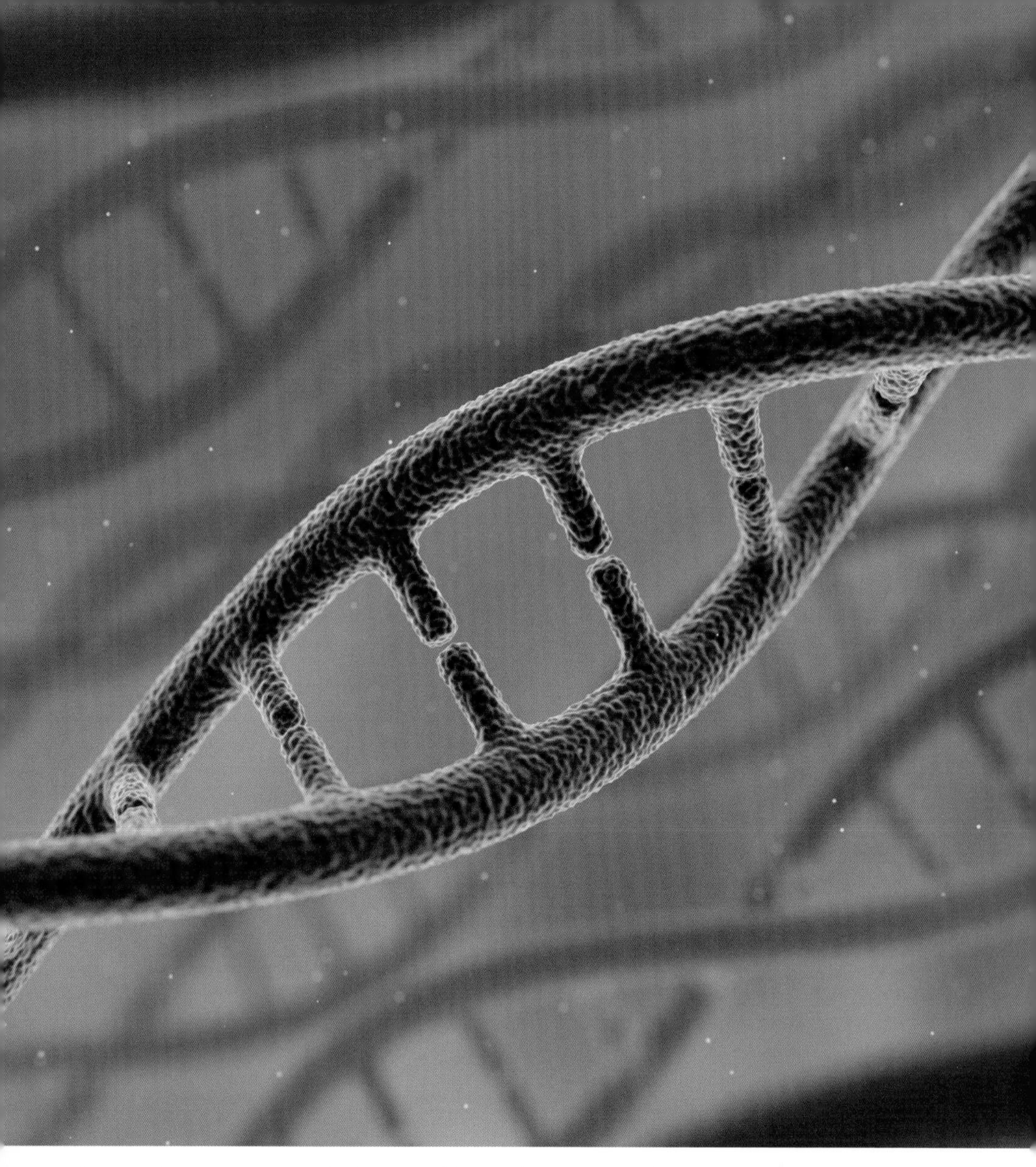

Researchers have found strong evidence that autism has a basis in a person's DNA. Individual genes have been linked to the disorder.

the brain develops. And because autism tends to run in families, scientists know that genes play an important role in autism, too.

Studies show that the odds of having an autistic child are significantly greater for parents with autism. When just one

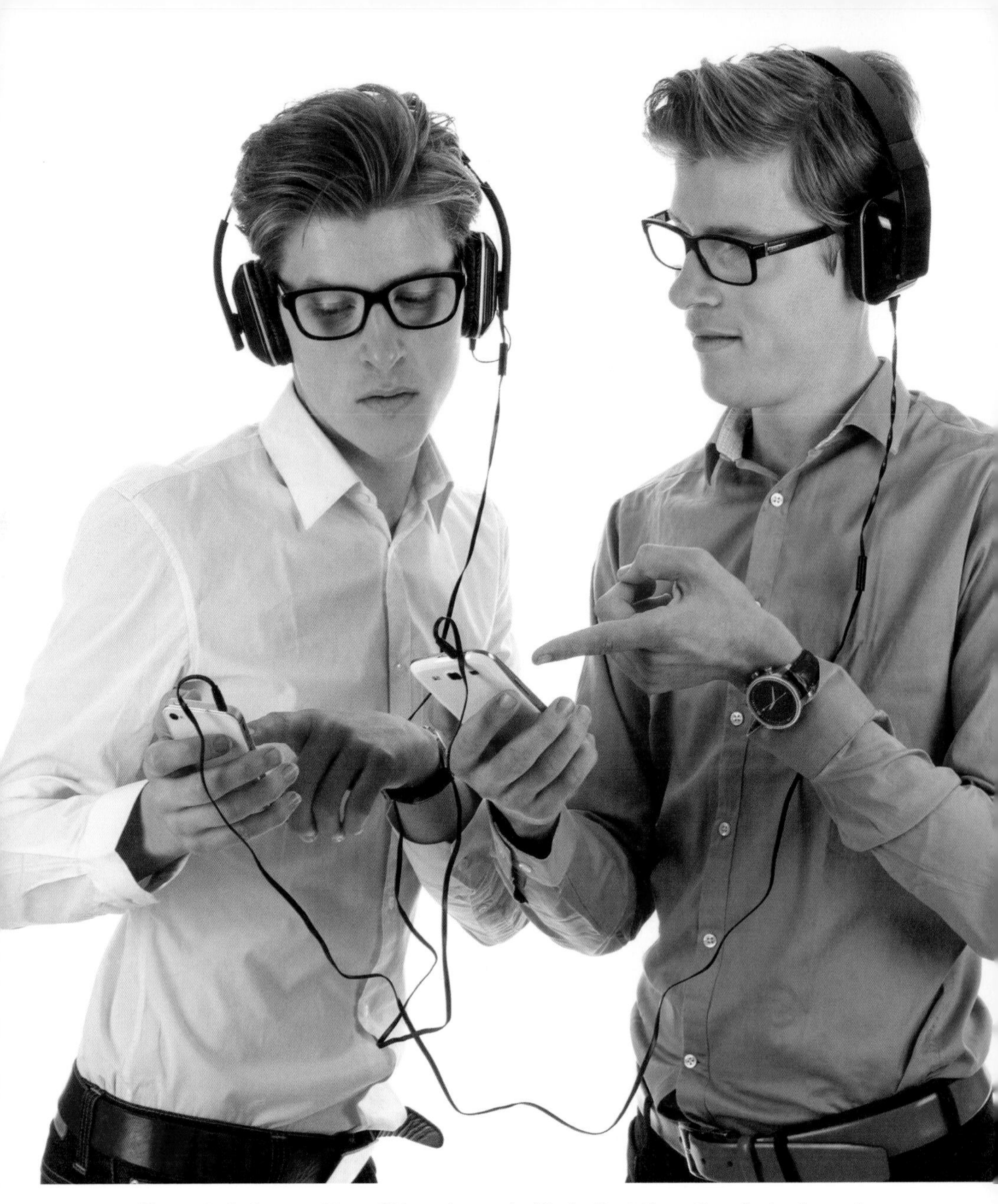

If one twin has autism, it is extremely likely that the other twin does, too. This suggests a strong genetic basis for the disorder.

parent has autistic traits, the likelihood of having a child with autism rises by more than 50 percent. When both parents have autistic traits, the odds increase by 85 percent.

Further evidence of the role of genes in autism comes from studies of fraternal and identical twins. Identical twins are the product of a single fertilized egg and so share 100 percent of their genes. Fraternal, or nonidentical, twins share only 50 percent of their genes because they come from two different fertilized eggs. According to the CDC, if one fraternal twin has autism, then the other twin has a roughly 31 percent chance of being autistic, too. But in the case of identical twins, the chance is as high as 95 percent. That's the highest correlation for any cognitive disorder.

Although it's clear that autism has a strong genetic basis, experts say there's no single gene or set of genes that causes the condition. Not all cases of autism involve the same genetic mutations, or alterations in DNA. And there don't seem to be any genetic mutations that always cause autism whenever they are present. Instead, scientists say, different patterns of genetic variations combine to produce the wide spectrum of symptoms observed among autistic people.

So far, hundreds of different genes have been found to be associated with autism. Some of these are linked to a single mutation. One example is the gene mutation that produces fragile X syndrome, a genetic disorder that causes intellectual disabilities. About one-third of people with fragile X also have autism. But autistic people with the fragile X gene mutation account for only a small fraction of all autism cases. Collectively, all the currently known single-gene mutations linked to autism are thought to explain only about 5 percent of all cases of autism.

In the majority of other cases, according to experts, autism involves a constellation of different gene traits. One study by researchers at the Hospital for Sick Children in Toronto, Canada, found that people with autism may have dozens of separate genetic mutations associated with their symptoms. Many of these genes have minor effects on their own and are even found in the general population. In combination with other genes, however, they increase a person's susceptibility to autism.

FACTORING IN THE ENVIRONMENT

Even when there is a very strong genetic basis for a disorder, the genes a person inherits are just one variable in a very complex process. Genetic inheritance may increase or decrease a person's risk of developing a particular condition. But whether and how it actually develops often depend on many nongenetic factors, including environmental conditions that act as triggers. Environmental conditions can affect how the brain develops at different stages and alter its biochemistry. They can influence how genes are expressed, or which parts of a person's DNA get switched on or off. They can even damage a person's genetic code, introducing new mutations not inherited from one's parents.

The environmental contribution to autism is not well understood, but there is growing support for the view that certain conditions in a developing fetus's prenatal environment may be significant risk factors for autism. For example, exposure in the womb to prescription drugs used to treat a range of conditions—from epilepsy to stomach ulcers—has been associated with increased risk of autism.

So has prenatal exposure to viral and bacterial infections.

Autism and Vaccines: A Debunked Theory

In 1998, British doctor Andrew Wakefield published a paper in a prestigious medical journal claiming to have discovered a link between autism and the measles, mumps, and rubella (MMR) vaccine—a routine vaccination given to millions of children around the world every year. Since then, the alleged link between vaccines and autism has been thoroughly debunked by scientists. And Wakefield's own research was found to be fraudulent. The journal later retracted his paper, and Wakefield was stripped of his medical license. Still, his work unleashed a growing anti-vaccination movement with devastating consequences.

Peter Hotez, a doctor at Baylor College of Medicine and father of an autistic daughter, says that the anti-vaccine movement doesn't just harm public health by eroding protections against dangerous diseases. It also hurts the autism cause itself by distracting from the real issues. "Not only are they putting kids in danger, it's doing something else. It's taking the oxygen out of an initiative to support kids with autism," he says. "Anytime autism is discussed at a high level, it's all about vaccines. Nobody focuses on what kids really need."

Quoted in Laura Beil, "Peter Hotez vs. Measles and the Anti-Vaccination Movement," Texas Monthly, *November 22, 2017. www.texasmonthly.com.*

Studies indicate that mothers who develop a viral infection such as rubella, also known as German measles, during the first trimester of pregnancy are roughly three times more likely to have a child with autism. Mothers with bacterial infections during the second trimester also appear to have an elevated risk, as do women with immune disorders. Scientists hypothesize that prenatal exposure to the antibodies produced by the mother's immune system may alter brain development in the growing fetus.

Chemicals and toxins in the environment are also thought to play a potentially important role. These include the chemical compounds in air pollution and pesticides, heavy metals such as lead and mercury, and hormone-disrupting compounds used to make plastic, such as bisphenol A (BPA). Excessive prenatal exposure to such chemicals can affect brain development in the growing fetus and even damage parts of the genetic code. "The weight of evidence is beginning to suggest that mothers' exposures during pregnancy may play a role in the development of autism spectrum disorders," says Kim Harley, an environmental health researcher at the University of California, Berkeley, School of Public Health.[22]

The exact role that such environmental factors play is still unclear, but experts say it is likely to be complex—like everything else about autism. "There are so many factors that likely contribute to the origins of autism," says Leonardo Trasande of the New York University School of Medicine. "It's impossible to point to any one factor for any one child."[23]

"The weight of evidence is beginning to suggest that mothers' exposures during pregnancy may play a role in the development of autism spectrum disorders."[22]

—Environmental health researcher Kim Harley

CHAPTER THREE

What Is Life like with Autism?

Advances in research are leading to new insights into the possible neurological, genetic, and environmental mechanisms behind autism. These findings are undoubtedly important—identifying different subtypes of autism and their causes and risk factors could allow researchers to find better treatments and interventions. "We can pursue individualized approaches and make a lot more progress in developing new treatments," explains University of Missouri professor David Beversdorf.[24]

But while working out the science of autism is important, so is finding concrete ways to improve the daily lives of people across the spectrum. And many autism advocates say that not enough resources are being applied to this goal. Of the more than $364 million spent on autism research in the United States in 2016, only 5 percent went toward studies focused on

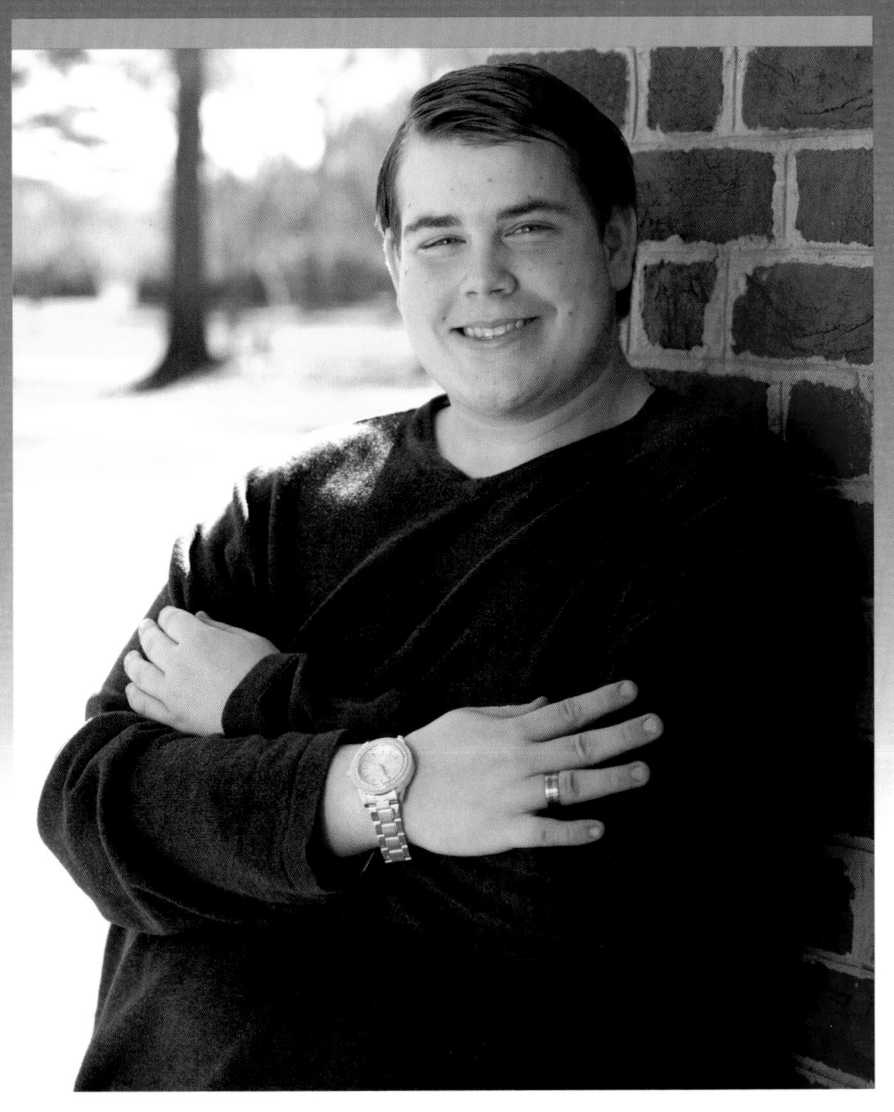

People with autism can live happy, full lives. Advocates believe more funding is needed to give these people the support they need to make this possible.

improving services. Just 2 percent went to researching how autism affects people across their lifespan. By comparison, approximately 60 percent went to theoretical research on biological causes and risk factors for autism.

Autism and Co-occurring Conditions

One of the challenges of living with autism is that it often comes with other accompanying physical or mental health conditions. These are called comorbid or co-occurring conditions. More than 95 percent of autistic children have at least one co-occurring condition. Fifty percent of all people with autism have at least four such conditions.

One of the most common comorbid conditions is attention-deficit/hyperactivity disorder (ADHD), which affects up to half of all children and teens with autism. People with ADHD have problems staying focused on tasks and controlling their impulses. Other conditions that frequently occur alongside autism are sleep disorders, allergies, and gastrointestinal disorders, including chronic—or recurring—problems with abdominal pain, constipation, and diarrhea.

Up to one-third of people with autism have epilepsy, a neurological disorder that causes seizures in the brain. The risk of having seizures tends to increase during puberty, possibly because of hormonal changes in the body. Many people on the spectrum also struggle with mood disorders, including depression and anxiety. Up to 40 percent of children and teens on the autism spectrum have an anxiety disorder, and up to 30 percent suffer from depression.

To help people on the spectrum live life to the fullest, more needs to be invested in services and support programs, autism advocates say. And more research is needed on the evolving issues that autistic people face over a lifetime—from childhood to adolescence to adulthood. "The challenges faced by people with autism change and evolve, and perhaps they are different at an older age—but they don't disappear," says Mathieu Vaillancourt, a writer and policy analyst with autism.[25]

DROPPING THE BALL

Because autism develops early in life, it is often thought of as a childhood condition. From the issues featured in news stories to the research that gets funded, public attention tends to focus almost exclusively on young children. But autism is a lifelong condition, and the increase in the numbers of children being diagnosed with autism means a growing number of teens and adults are living with autism. In the decade following 2019, an estimated 500,000 teens diagnosed with autism will enter adulthood, according to the autism advocacy organization Autism Speaks. Currently, few resources are in place to deal with the distinct needs and realities of these young people, experts say. "We are, on the whole, unprepared to help them function to their true potential," says Susan White, a professor at the University of Alabama.[26] Paul Shattuck, director of the Life Course Outcomes Research Program at Drexel University, concurs. "We're expending a lot of effort for very young children with autism, but as a society we kind of drop the ball once these young people become young adults," he says.[27]

> "We're expending a lot of effort for very young children with autism, but as a society we kind of drop the ball once these young people become young adults."[27]
>
> *—Paul Shattuck, director of the Life Course Outcomes Research Program at Drexel University*

TEENS ON THE SPECTRUM

Adolescence tends to be a confusing and stressful time for teens. For young people with autism, these years can be especially challenging. Adjusting to more complex school schedules and to changing roles and expectations can be difficult for people on the spectrum, who typically have trouble coping with changes and transitions. And at a stage in life when peer relationships are especially important, autistic teens may struggle to fit in socially.

Many people with autism have behaviors that make them stand out as different. They may have trouble making eye contact, engage in repetitive motions such as hand flapping, or talk obsessively about a single topic. They may miss—or misinterpret—the subtle cues that govern social interactions, such as tone of voice, facial expressions, or body language. "Autistic people don't pick up on those cues," autistic author Kamran Nazeer explains. "They might be noticing instead the pattern of coals in the fireplace or the details on the lamp and so on."[28]

Standing out as different can lead to social exclusion. Studies show that almost one-third of young adults with autism never receive social phone calls, hang out with friends, or get invited to activities. "Difficulty navigating the terrain of friendships and social interaction is a hallmark feature of autism," says Dr. Shattuck. "Nonetheless, many people with autism do indeed have a social appetite. They yearn for connection with others. We need better ways of supporting positive social connection and of

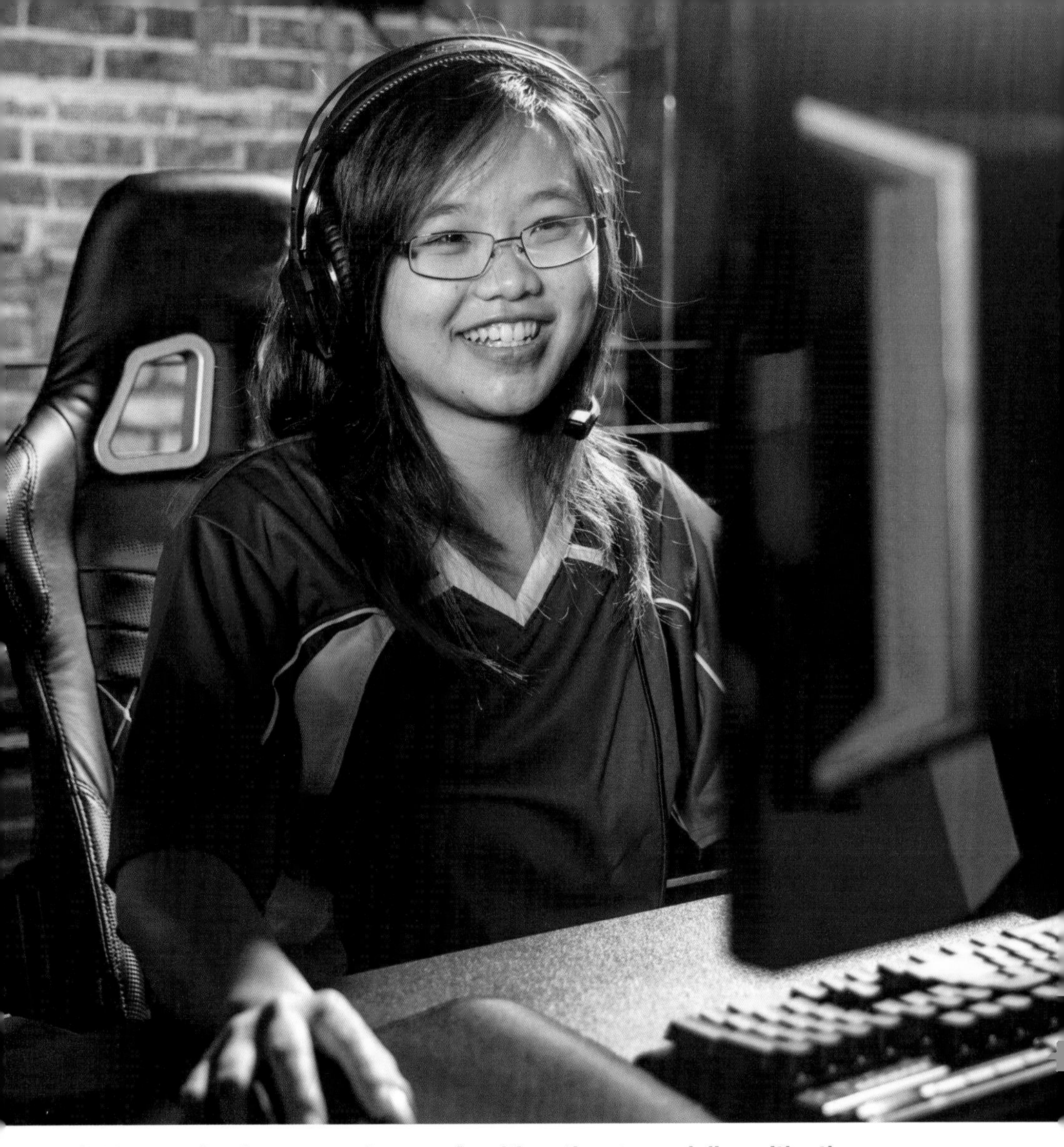

Online gaming is one way for people with autism to socialize with others. This may be easier than socializing in person.

preventing social isolation."[29] Dr. Brad Ferguson, a neuroscientist at the University of Missouri Thompson Center for Autism and Neurodevelopmental Disorders, notes that some people connect in nontraditional ways. He says, "Many individuals with autism spectrum disorder yearn to connect with others, but perhaps not

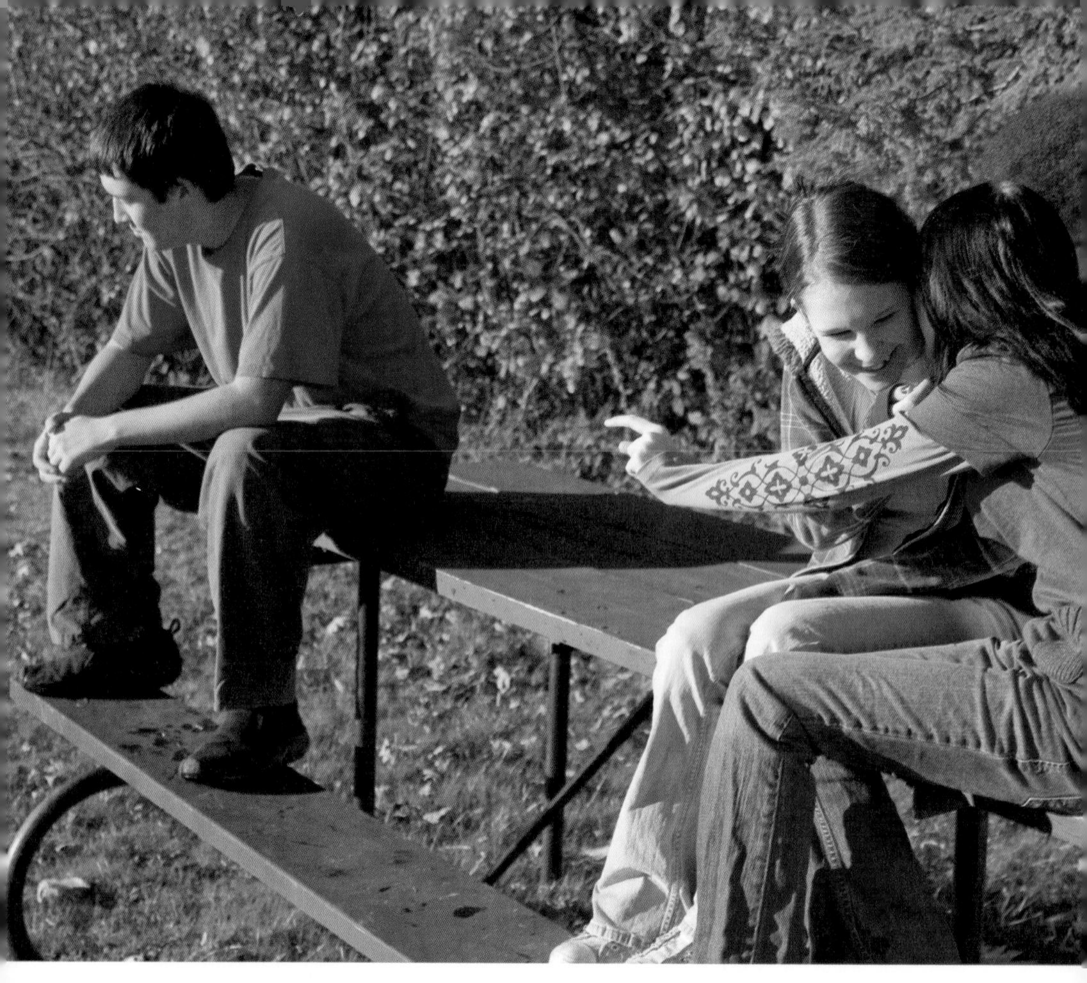

Bullying of people with autism is common. Those with autism can find people with similar interests to help them connect to others.

in traditional ways. I see many adolescents with autism spectrum disorder that have lots of online friends that they talk to daily over the internet while playing video games, and we may miss these interactions with traditional questionnaires and assessments in a laboratory setting."[30]

In addition to struggling with social skills, autistic children and teens are at increased risk of being bullied. Lillian, a parent of an autistic teen, says her son was called names and teased relentlessly in middle school. "All of the bullying can be tied back to his spectrum behaviors: his lack of focus, his pickiness about certain things, his obsessive fixations on Superman or super heroes, and non-social behavior in general," she says. "He doesn't know how to socialize, and nothing we have tried has really helped."[31]

Although social interaction and communication can be challenging for people on the spectrum, many autistic teens do enjoy meaningful friendships and a satisfying social life. Building on shared interests is a good way to connect with others, advocates say. And joining a club or organization can provide ready-made opportunities for socialization.

For Temple Grandin, for example, a passion for horses and rockets became a way to make friends—and escape bullies. "When I was in high school being teased by other kids, I was miserable. The only place I was not teased was during horseback riding and model rocket club," she writes in her book *Thinking in Pictures*. "The students who were interested in these special interests were not the kids who did the teasing. These activities were a shared interest."[32]

FACING THE "CLIFF"

Autistic teens can face many challenges during adolescence, but one of the biggest may be preparing for the transition to adulthood. Because autism can affect the brain's ability to process information, many people on the spectrum struggle to keep up with the realities of adult life, such as paying bills, staying healthy, getting a job, and finding a place to live. Yet after graduation, young people with autism have a much harder time finding help. While in school, autistic kids are guaranteed access by law to special education services that provide vital support. Once they turn twenty-one, however, these support services abruptly drop away—a period of life experts refer to as "the cliff."

"When teens exit high school, they fall off what is called the services cliff," Dr. Shattuck says. "It becomes much more difficult to find help and services once kids age out of eligibility for special education."[33] Although some community programs are available, there are not enough of them in place to serve everyone who needs them. As a result, many young adults with autism find themselves in limbo after high school, with few resources to help smooth the transition to adult life. In fact, studies show that some 39 percent of autistic young adults receive no services at all. Most of the rest make do with very limited services.

"When teens exit high school, they fall off what is called the services cliff. It becomes much more difficult to find help and services once kids age out of eligibility for special education."[33]

—Paul Shattuck, director of the Life Course Outcomes Research Program at Drexel University

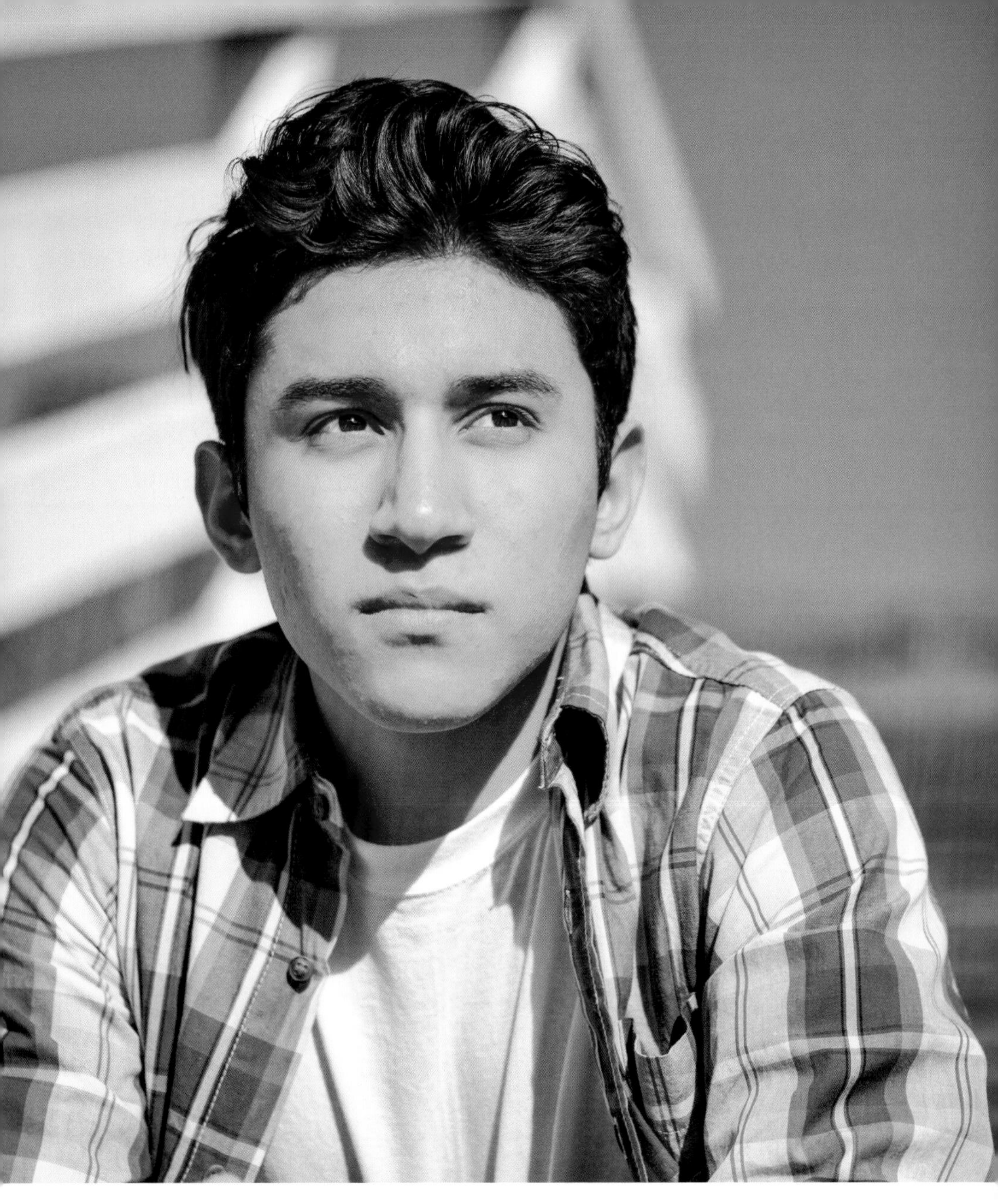

Social isolation can be a challenge for people with autism. Advocates are pushing for more social services and community programs to help these people.

This lack of support can have far-ranging impacts on quality of life, affecting access to health care, career training, and educational opportunities. Compared with people with other disabilities, autistic adults are roughly three times more likely to be socially isolated. They are also significantly less likely to live independently, or outside of the family home, and significantly more likely to be unemployed. Two years after high school, only 50 percent of young people with autism are employed or enrolled in college—a lower rate than young people with other disabilities, including learning disabilities, speech impairments, or intellectual disabilities.

Kiely Law says that her twenty-four-year-old son, Isaac, is typical of many young adults on the spectrum. Since graduating from high school, he spends

"Islands of Genius"

Along with disabilities, autism sometimes comes with remarkable abilities. An estimated one in ten people on the autism spectrum have a condition known as savant syndrome, derived from the French verb *savoir*, meaning "to know." This is a rare condition in which people have cognitive impairments combined with extreme talents in a specific area. Researcher Darold Treffert, who studies the phenomenon, describes savant skills as "islands of genius" within an overall handicap. Some autistic savants can perform extraordinary feats of mental calculation, such as computing prime numbers at lightning speed or instantly calculating the day of the week for any past or future date. Others have special abilities in fields such as music, art, and mathematics, often combined with an astonishing memory. For example, Stephen Wiltshire, a British autistic savant, has been called a "human camera" because of his uncanny ability to draw cityscapes in intricate detail from memory. Rex Lewis-Clack, who is both blind and autistic, can play a piece of music on the piano from start to finish after hearing it only once.

Darold A. Treffert, "The Savant Syndrome: An Extraordinary Condition," Philosophical Transactions of the Royal Society B: Biological Sciences, *364, no. 1522 (2009): 1351–1357.*

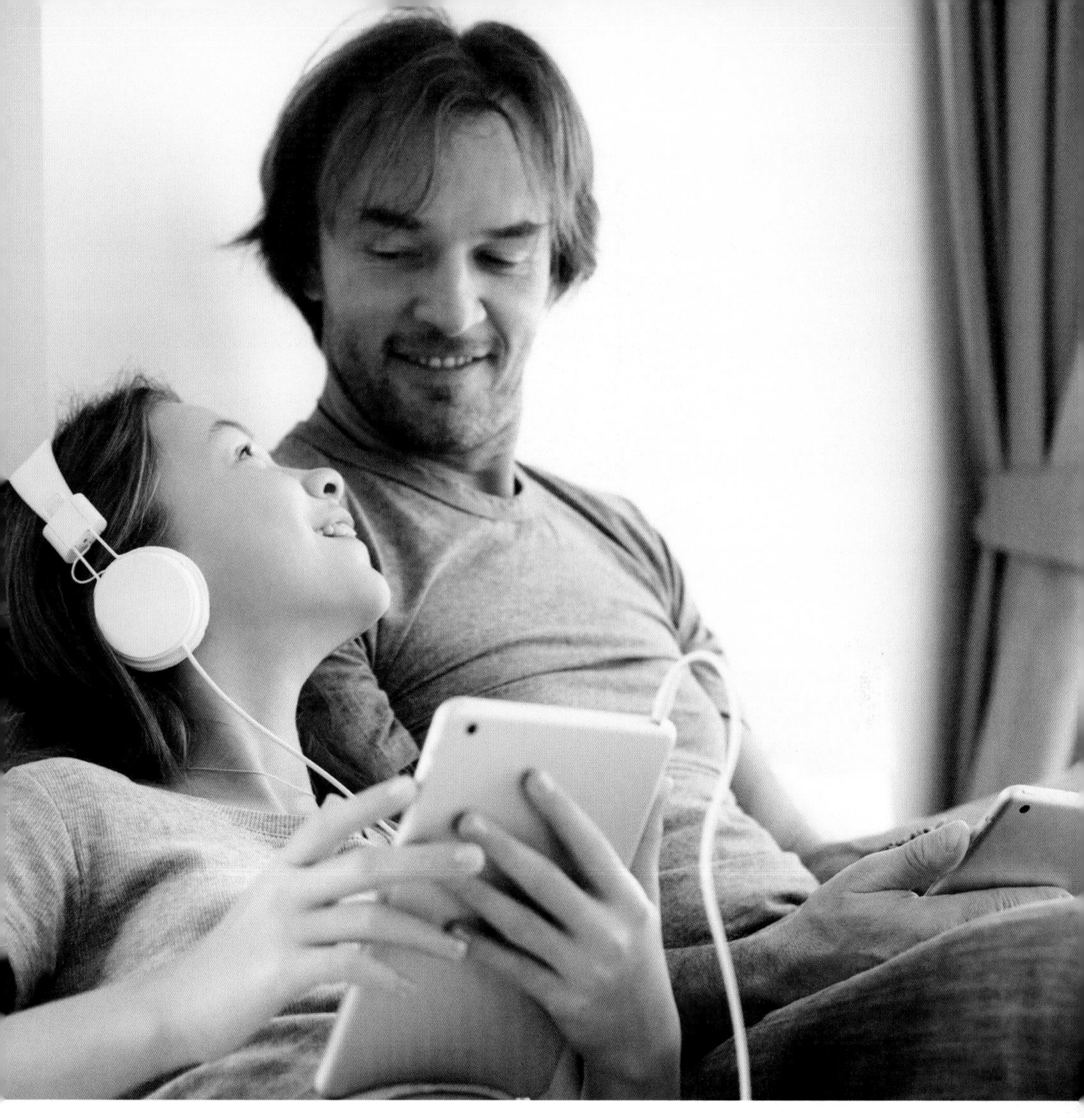

Finding and focusing on the strengths of a person with autism can be the key to a successful transition to adulthood. Parents can start discussing this with their children at a young age.

most of his time alone in his room. He doesn't take classes or have a job. "I think one of his challenges is that, like many adults with autism, he has some extremely narrow interests," she says. "The opportunities that exist don't fit what he's interested in. And if you have difficulties relating to other people, and with social skills, and difficulties with transportation, it just snowballs."[34]

BUILDING ON STRENGTHS

Paradoxically, experts say that teens able to do more things independently—like Isaac—may have a tougher time navigating the transition to adulthood than those with intellectual disabilities. In large part, this is because intellectually disabled adults have access to a greater range of services. Teens with average or above intelligence have needs that are less visible and so are more likely to be overlooked. They may have higher expectations and ambitions for themselves but a harder time finding support to help them reach their goals. The gap between their goals and their reality can cause depression and anxiety.

Given how difficult the transition to adulthood can be, experts say that one of the best thing teens and their families can do is plan ahead. "Young adults with autism really want to be able to socialize and succeed in higher education, but sometimes they don't know how to go about doing that," says Nancy Cheak-Zamora, an autism researcher at the University of Missouri. "Caregivers need to start saying to their children at the age of 12 or 13, 'What do you want to do? We've got 5 years, so let's make a plan.'"[35]

Building on strengths is also key, advocates say. Discussions of autism often focus exclusively on the deficits, or weaknesses, associated with autism. Yet many people with autism have superior skills in other areas, such as exceptional pattern recognition skills, an excellent memory, or the ability to focus for a long time on tasks requiring great attention to detail. Helping teens on the spectrum tap into their talents is a crucial step on the path to a fulfilling life. "If you really want to prepare kids to participate in the mainstream of life, then you have to do more than accommodate their deficits," Temple Grandin says. "You have to figure out ways to exploit their strengths."[36]

"If you really want to prepare kids to participate in the mainstream of life, then you have to do more than accommodate their deficits. You have to figure out ways to exploit their strengths."[36]

—Temple Grandin

CHAPTER FOUR

How Is Autism Managed?

When Bruno Youn was diagnosed with autism at the age of four, he was largely nonverbal. He could parrot words that he heard but couldn't communicate his own thoughts or feelings. He struggled to follow directions and to interact with others. He needed an aide with him at all times at school. His mother hired speech and behavioral therapists to help him with his language, motor, and social skills, but worried that he would never talk, hold down a job, or get married. "I was dreaming he would be in good enough shape to work at a grocery store," she says.[37]

Today, Bruno has more than defied his mother's fears. In 2019, the twenty-two-year-old landed a great job with a tech startup after graduating from Claremont McKenna College, a selective liberal arts college in California. He had been an honors student with a 3.8 GPA. He took on leadership roles and had an

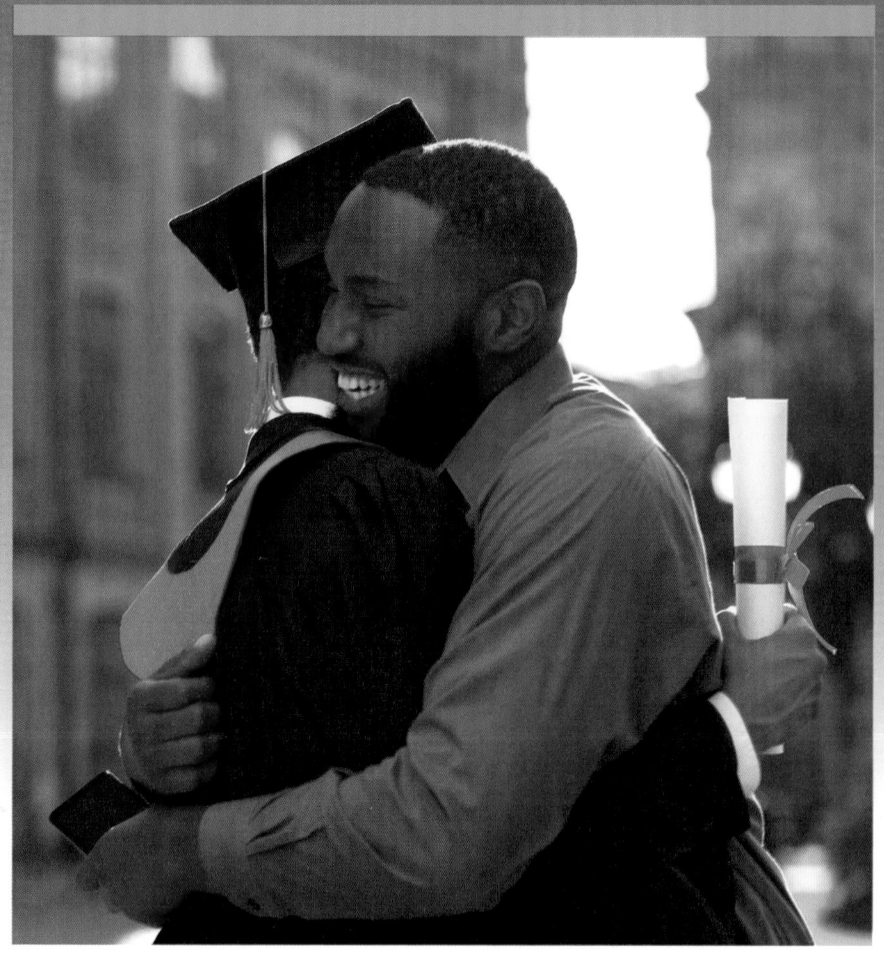

With support from friends and family, many people with autism can achieve academic success. Still, they are challenged by their autism symptoms in daily life.

active social life. And at graduation, Bruno was chosen to deliver the student commencement speech in front of an audience of hundreds.

Bruno's autism hasn't gone away. Socializing still doesn't come naturally to him. Too much time in a group setting leaves him exhausted. He has to constantly think about how to act, mentally reminding himself to make more eye contact, for example, or to talk less mechanically. But Bruno has achieved successes his younger self could never have imagined. "I have left behind me a trail of broken stereotypes," Youn said in his commencement speech.[38]

EARLY INTERVENTION

Not everyone with autism can be expected to be as successful as Bruno, just as not all nonautistic people turn out to be high achievers. But the right support and accommodations, advocates say, can help all autistic people—wherever they lie on the spectrum—to reach their full potential. Early intervention is an important step in that direction, experts say. To that end, many researchers are making a major push to find ways to diagnose autism at earlier and earlier ages.

The hope is that early diagnosis will allow for therapy to start early, taking advantage of the young brain's plasticity, or ability to "rewire" itself by forming new patterns of neural connections. "The reason why we are focusing so much on early diagnosis is that it is our hope that by intervening early, we can capitalize on still tremendous brain plasticity that is present in the first, second, third year of life," explains Katarzyna Chawarska, a professor of child psychiatry at Yale University's School of Medicine.[39]

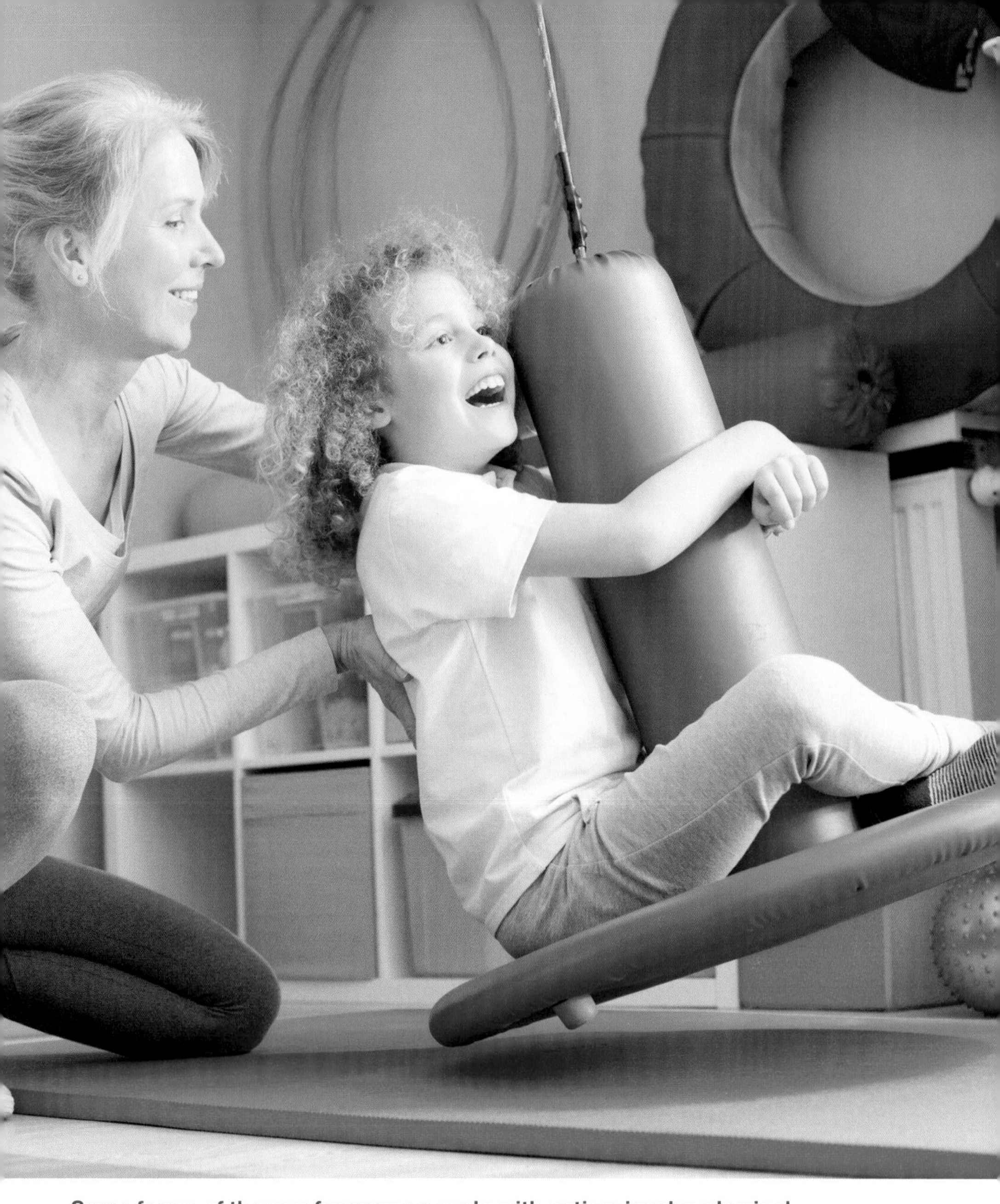

Some forms of therapy for young people with autism involve physical exercise. This is meant to help develop motor skills, strength, and balance.

For example, researchers hope that early treatments could tweak the developmental trajectory of the brain so as to weaken the effect of intellectual disabilities or strengthen communication

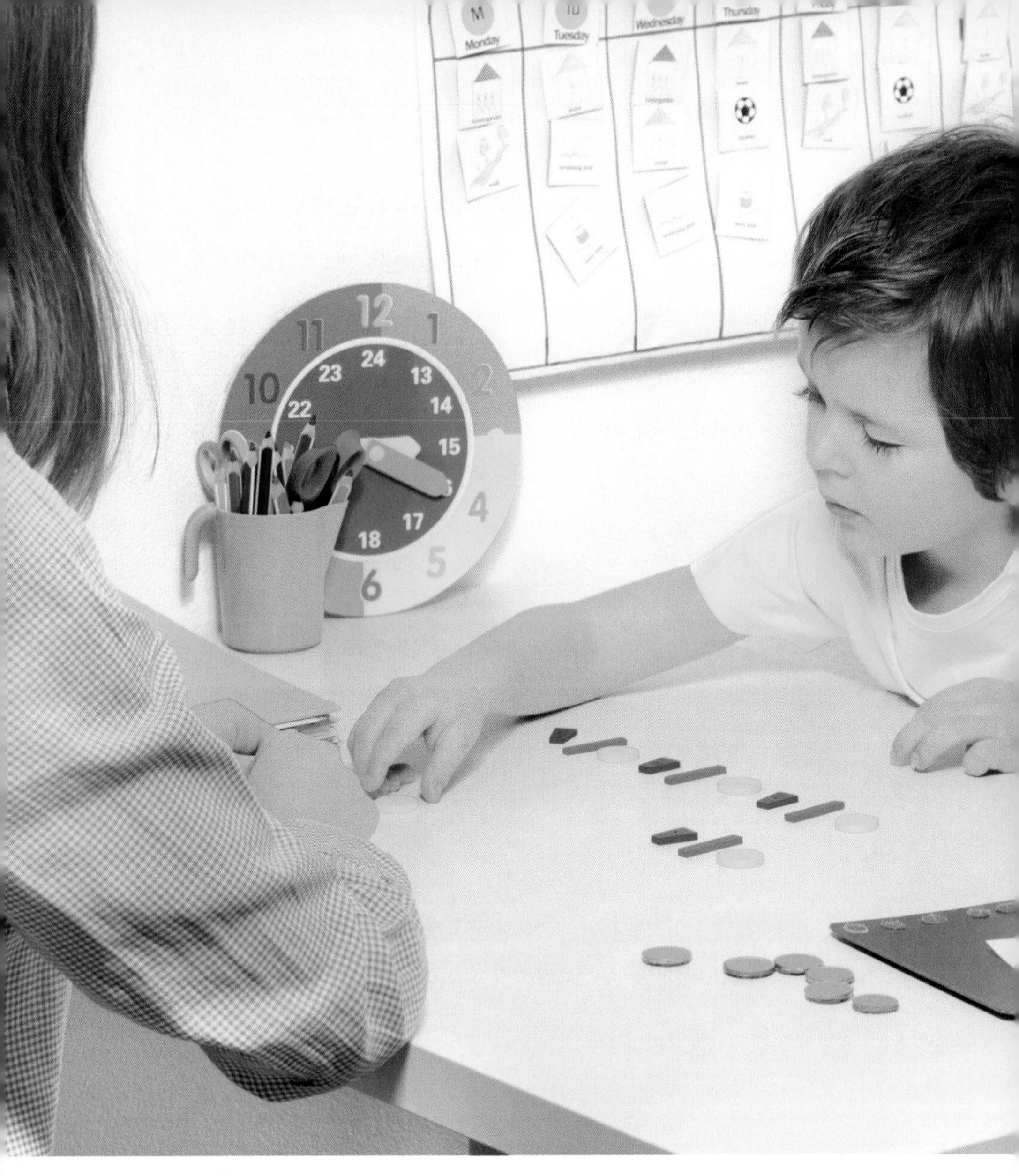

Applied behavior analysis (ABA) is a common way for therapists to work with children with autism. It may involve tasks such as sorting objects.

and social skills. Early intervention could also allow doctors to get a head start on addressing co-occurring conditions that compound the symptoms of autism, such as epilepsy, gastrointestinal problems, or ADHD.

But while the consensus is that early intervention is ideal, experts agree that therapy can help at any age. The brain's plasticity starts declining in the teenage years, but it never disappears altogether. "Treatment can have effects even very late," says Kevin Pelphrey, also of Yale University. "It's not a lost cause at all."[40]

> "The reason why we are focusing so much on early diagnosis is that it is our hope that by intervening early, we can capitalize on still tremendous brain plasticity that is present in the first, second, third year of life"[39]
>
> —*Child psychiatry professor Katarzyna Chawarska*

THERAPIES FOR AUTISM

So far, the most common treatments for autism are therapy based. Unlike medications, which target the underlying physiology of an illness, therapy-based interventions focus on a person's behaviors and thinking processes. The emphasis is on learning skills and working through emotional, social, and behavioral challenges with one-on-one help from a trained professional.

For autism, the most well-established type of therapy is applied behavior analysis (ABA), a method first introduced in the 1960s by Norwegian American psychologist Ole Ivar Lovaas. ABA is based on the idea of positive reinforcement: the therapist breaks down tasks and behaviors into small steps, and the person is rewarded for each step completed along the way.

The Power of Technology

For many people on the autism spectrum, technology is a life-changing tool. The internet can provide an important social outlet for people who struggle with face-to-face interaction, offering an environment where problems with eye contact are not visible.

Technology can even give a voice to those otherwise unable to communicate—as with Carly Fleischmann. Diagnosed with severe symptoms of autism at the age of two, Carly is unable to speak and struggles with motor skills. Learning to type on a keyboard at the age of ten, however, was a breakthrough moment for the native of Toronto, Canada. Now Carly uses a handheld tablet to communicate her thoughts and feelings. Text-to-speech technology translates her typed words into speech.

In her twenties, Carly became the first nonverbal person to host a talk show, interviewing celebrities on her YouTube show *Speechless with Carly Fleischmann*. "Technology has allowed me to communicate, learn social skills, implement relaxing techniques and played a crucial part in helping me [learn] how to spell," Carly says. "To me, technology is the key to unlocking autism."

Quoted in Callie Carmichael, "How Tablets Helped Unlock One Girl's Voice," CNN, *November 14, 2012. www.cnn.com.*

The goal is to encourage desirable skills—such as making eye contact or learning to spell—and discourage problematic behaviors, such as self-injury or excessive stimming.

Some critics worry that ABA is too tough on kids. The therapy can involve up to forty hours a week of intensive one-on-one work. Some also object to what they see as the overarching goal of ABA—to force children with autism to suppress their real selves in order to appear more "normal" and fit into society.

Despite the controversies, however, ABA is still considered the gold standard of autism therapies. A considerable amount of research points to a track record of success in helping autistic kids to function better. "There is a lot of good clinical evidence that it is effective in helping little kids learn new skills and can appropriately intervene with behaviors or characteristics that may interfere with progress," says Susan Levy, a doctor with the Center for Autism Research at the Children's Hospital of Philadelphia.[41]

Many kids on the spectrum benefit from other types of therapy as well, including speech therapy and occupational therapy, which helps with skills such as handwriting, motor skills, or daily living skills. There is also some evidence that alternative therapies using music and dance can also enhance communication skills and social interaction in people with autism. "Parents report that their children with autism enjoy musical activities and show more positive interactions with others through greater eye contact, smiling and speaking after engaging in a dance and music program," says Anjana Bhat, a professor in the physical therapy department at the University of Delaware.[42]

"Parents report that their children with autism enjoy musical activities and show more positive interactions with others through greater eye contact, smiling and speaking after engaging in a dance and music program."[42]

—Physical therapy professor Anjana Bhat

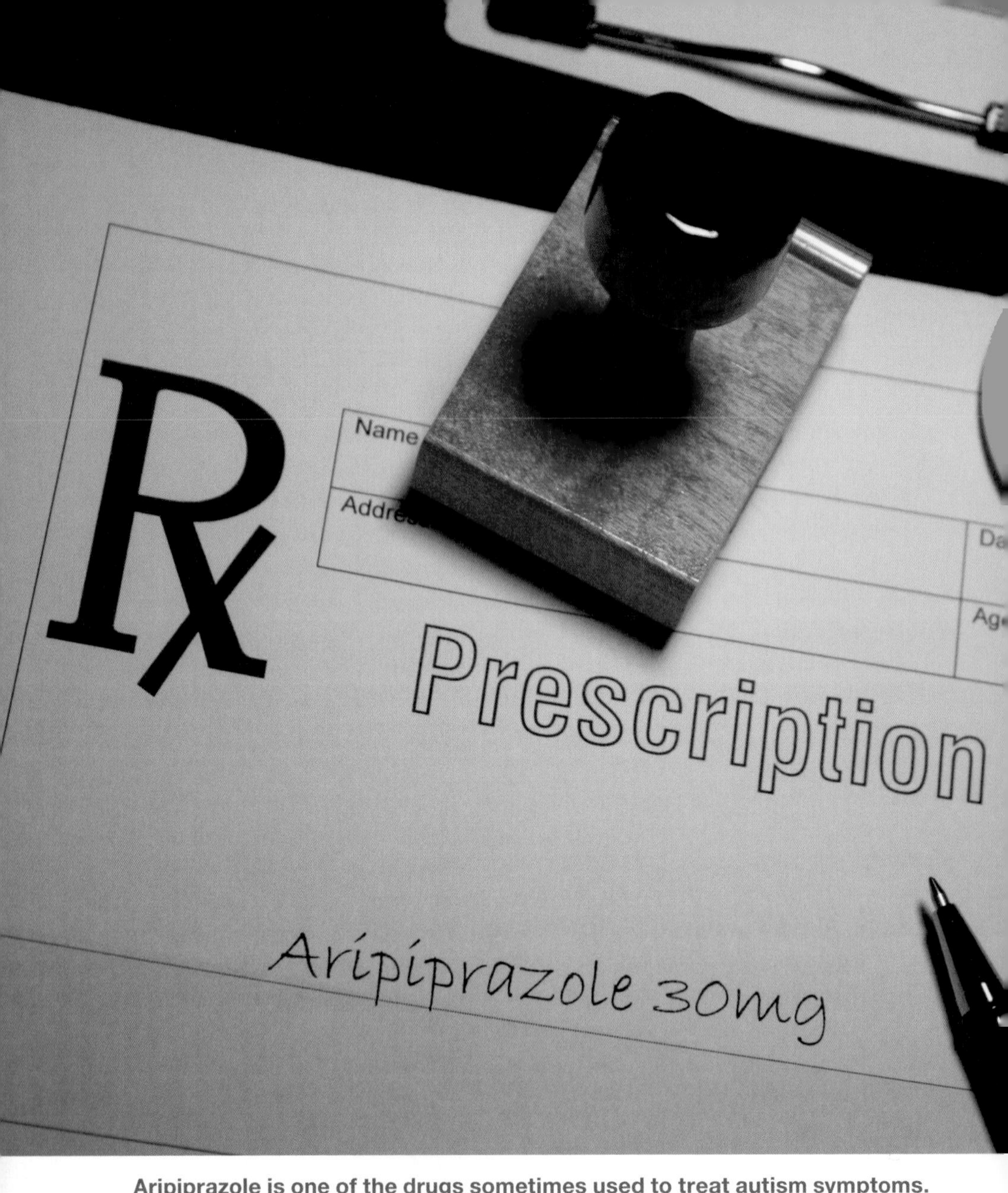

Aripiprazole is one of the drugs sometimes used to treat autism symptoms. It is also sold under the brand name Abilify.

NO MAGIC BULLET

Behavioral interventions such as ABA and other types of therapies can make a big difference in autistic kids' lives. However, such therapies are not considered to be a cure for autism. Neither are any of the other treatments currently available for people on the spectrum.

Some of the comorbid conditions that commonly occur alongside autism, such as anxiety, depression, sleep disorders, and epilepsy, can be treated with medicines approved by the Food and Drug Administration (FDA). There are also two FDA-approved drugs—risperidone and aripiprazole—that can help reduce agitation and aggression in autistic children. These medicines can help control explosive tantrums and meltdowns. They can also relieve the self-injurious behaviors that afflict almost 28 percent of

Risky Business

In the absence of any known medical treatments for autism, many parents turn to alternative therapies, or treatments outside the boundaries of conventional medicine. Up to 54 percent of autistic children receive such alternative forms of treatment, experts say. Vitamin supplements are among the most common, including supplementation with vitamin B12, vitamin D, and fish oil. Special diets have also been touted as potential remedies.

There is little evidence that any of these alternative therapies are effective. Moreover, the FDA warns that such treatments need to be used with caution and always with the approval of a doctor. Some supplements, including high doses of certain vitamins, can have risky side effects. And some of the treatments peddled to desperate parents are downright dangerous.

For example, chelation therapy claims to cure autism by stripping heavy metals, such as mercury, from the body. In reality, however, there is no evidence that it works, and the risky procedure can cause serious health problems—even death. Another dangerous procedure involves giving children chlorine dioxide, a form of bleach. "It can lead to kidney damage and kidney failure," says Daniel Brooks, medical director of the Banner Poison and Drug Information Center in Phoenix, Arizona.

Brandy Zadrozny, "Parents Are Poisoning Their Children with Bleach to 'Cure' Autism," NBC News, *May 21, 2019. www.nbcnews.com.*

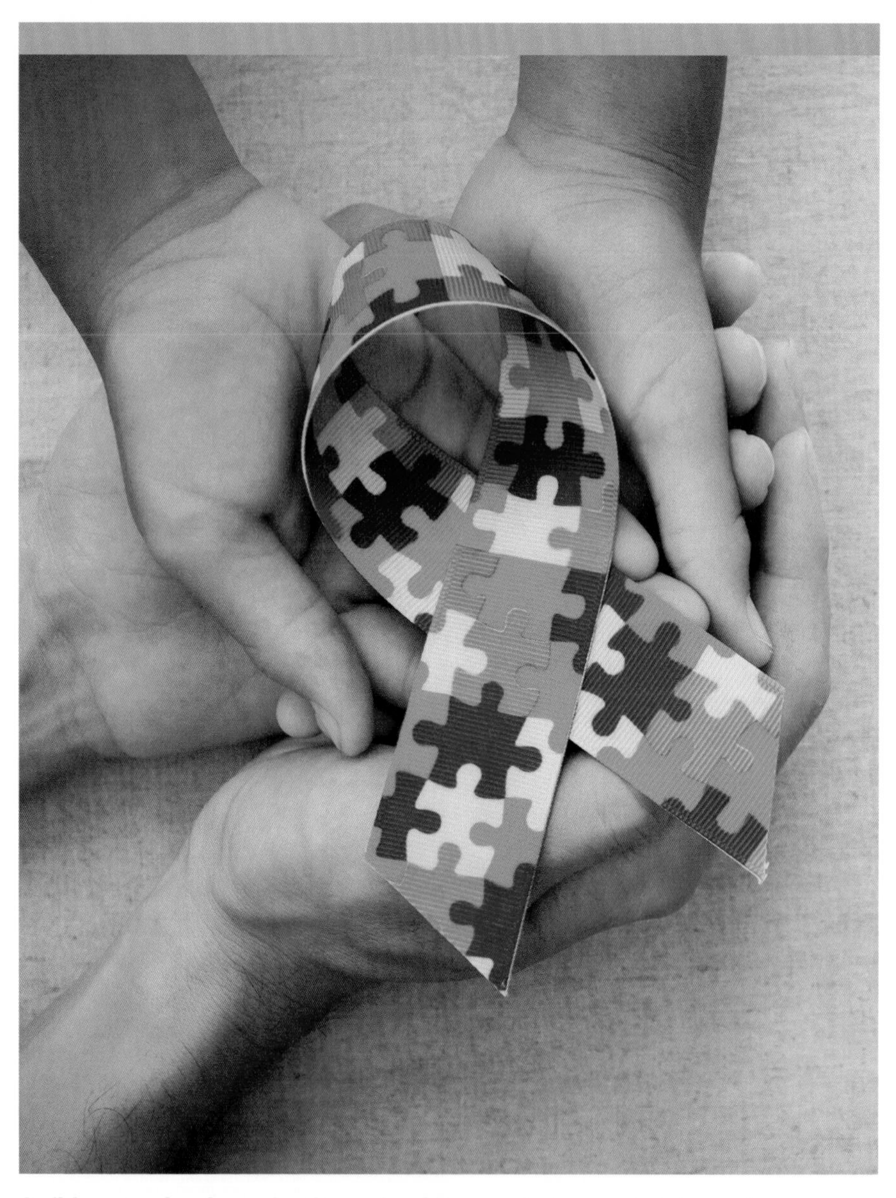

A ribbon made of puzzle pieces is often used as a symbol for autism awareness. Created by the Autism Society, it represents the complexity and diversity of people with autism.

kids on the spectrum, such as head banging and arm biting. However, there are currently no FDA-approved medications that target the core symptoms of autism.

Research into potential medical treatments continues. For example, some scientists see promise in an experimental treatment called transcranial magnetic stimulation. This is a noninvasive procedure that involves stimulating parts of the brain with magnetic impulses to change how the brain cells function. Scientists are also investigating treatments using the hormone oxytocin—known as the "love hormone" because of its role in facilitating feelings of social attachment. Research is also underway on other drugs that may improve the social interaction aspects of autism.

But it's unlikely that any of these or other possible treatments will turn out to be a one-size-fits-all remedy for autism, researchers say. Just as there is no single autism gene, there is probably no straightforward cure for autism.

DIFFERENCE OR DISABILITY?

Some members of the autism community say that trying to cure autism is not an appropriate goal anyway. "We don't view autism as a disease to be cured, and we don't think it needs fixing," says Ari Ne'emen, an autism rights activist and cofounder of the Autistic Self Advocacy Network (ASAN), an organization that promotes autism acceptance and is run by autistic people.[43]

Ne'emen, who was diagnosed with Asperger's as a child, represents a growing trend within the autism community known as the neurodiversity movement. The term *neurodiversity* refers to the idea that there is a tremendous amount of variation in the way that human brains are wired. Autism, in this view, is just one manifestation of that neurological diversity—a difference that society should accept and accommodate, not a defect that needs to be prevented, treated, or cured. "If you're trying to get rid of autism, you're trying to get rid of us," says Julia Bascom, current president of ASAN.[44]

The neurodiversity movement has become controversial because some critics argue that the debate is dominated by people with milder symptoms—people who can vocally advocate for themselves precisely because they are less afflicted. In the process, critics say, less attention gets paid to the needs of people with severe autism—those who cannot speak for themselves.

"There's a wide abyss between someone who is very mildly impaired and someone who is really severely impaired with intellectual disability and all the different kinds of comorbid conditions that tend to cluster at that end of the spectrum," says Amy Lutz.[45] She's the mother of a twenty-year-old son with severe autistic traits, including self-harming behaviors.

Both sides, however, can agree on at least one goal: improving the lives of all people on the spectrum. To encompass the full breadth of that spectrum, there needs to be room made for both sides of the debate. Ultimately, autism can be both a disability and a difference, says psychologist Simon Baron-Cohen, an autism researcher at Cambridge University in the United Kingdom. "We need to find ways of alleviating the disability while respecting and valuing the difference."[46]

> "We need to find ways of alleviating the disability while respecting and valuing the difference."[46]
>
> *—Psychologist Simon Baron-Cohen*

Source Notes

Introduction: Struggling to Fit In

1. Temple Grandin, *Thinking in Pictures: My Life with Autism*. New York: Doubleday, 1995, pp. 62–64.

2. Grandin, *Thinking in Pictures*, p. 17.

3. Quoted in Oliver Sacks, "An Anthropologist on Mars," *New Yorker*, December 27, 1993. www.newyorker.com.

Chapter 1: What Is Autism?

4. Quoted in Emily L. Casanova and Manuel Casanova, *Defining Autism: A Guide to Brain, Biology, and Behavior*. Philadelphia, PA: Jessica Kingsley Publishers, 2018, p. 14.

5. Quoted in *In a Different Key: The Story of Autism*. New York: Crown Publishers, 2016, pp. 25–42.

6. Quoted in Andrew Solomon, *Far from the Tree: Parents, Children, and the Search for Identity*. New York: Scribner, 2012, p. 233.

7. Grandin, *Thinking in Pictures*, p. 34.

8. Quoted in Emily Willingham, "Spike in Autism Numbers Might Reflect Rise in Awareness," *Scientific American*, April 1, 2014. www.scientificamerican.com.

9. Quoted in Susan Scutti, "Autism Prevalence Increases: 1 in 59 US Children," *CNN*, April 26, 2018. www.cnn.com.

10. Solomon, *Far from the Tree*, p. 245.

11. Ido Kedar, "I Was Born Unable to Speak, and a Disputed Treatment Saved Me," *Wall Street Journal*, September 23, 2018. www.wsj.com.

12. Lorna Selfe, *Autism Spectrum Disorder: All That Matters.* New York: McGraw-Hill Education, 2014, p. 10.

Chapter 2: What Causes Autism?

13. Casanova and Casanova, *Defining Autism*, p. 21.

14. Quoted in Pam Belluck, "Study Finds That Brains with Autism Fail to Trim Synapses as They Develop," *New York Times*, August 21, 2014. www.nytimes.com.

15. Quoted in Tamara Bhandari, "In Autism, Too Many Brain Connections May Be at Root of Condition," *Washington University School of Medicine in St. Louis*, November 2, 2017. https://medicine.wustl.edu.

16. Casanova and Casanova, *Defining Autism*, p. 190.

17. Quoted in Solomon, *Far from the Tree*, p. 246.

18. Quoted in "EEG Signals Accurately Predict Autism as Early as 3 Months of Age," *Science Daily*, May 1, 2018. www.sciencedaily.com.

19. Quoted in John J. Pitney Jr., *The Politics of Autism: Navigating the Contested Spectrum*. Lanham, MD: Rowman & Littlefield, 2015, p. 36.

20. Temple Grandin, *The Autistic Brain: Thinking Across the Spectrum*. Boston: Houghton Mifflin Harcourt, 2013, p. 37.

21. Christian Jarrett, "Autism – Myth and Reality," *British Psychological Society*, October 2014. https://thepsychologist.bps.org.uk.

22. Quoted in Lindsey Konkel, "Autism Risk Higher near Pesticide-Treated Fields," *Scientific American*, June 23, 2014. www.scientificamerican.com.

23. Quoted in Perri Klass, "In Baby Teeth, Links Between Chemical Exposure in Pregnancy and Autism," *New York Times,* July 2, 2018. www.nytimes.com.

Source Notes Continued

Chapter 3: What Is Life like with Autism?

24. Quoted in "Link Found Between Neurotransmitter Imbalance, Brain Connectivity in Those with Autism," *Medical Xpress*, June 6, 2018. www.medicalxpress.com.

25. Mathieu Vaillancourt, "It's No Surprise that People with Autism Have a Low Life Expectancy. Our Needs as Adults Are Being Ignored," *Independent*, April 2, 2016. www.independent.co.uk.

26. Quoted in Teresa Watanabe, "He Couldn't Speak as a Child. Now This Autistic Student Is Giving a Commencement Address," *Los Angeles Times*, May 17, 2019. www.latimes.com.

27. Quoted in Jacqueline Stenson, "Why the Focus of Autism Research Is Shifting Away from Searching for a 'Cure,'" *NBC News*, September 22, 2019. www.nbcnews.com.

28. Quoted in "'We Want to Have Conversations, to Do the Things Everybody Else Does,'" *Guardian*, March 4, 2006. www.theguardian.com.

29. Quoted in Shaun Heasley, "Study: Nearly 1 in 3 with Autism Socially Isolated," *Disability Scoop*, May 8, 2013. www.disabilityscoop.com.

30. Dr. Brad Ferguson, Personal interview, February 15, 2020.

31. Quoted in Marina Sarris, "Families Face Autism Stigma, Isolation," *Interactive Autism Network*, February 4, 2016. www.iancommunity.org.

32. Grandin, *Thinking in Pictures*, p. 162.

33. Quoted in Stenson, "Why the Focus of Autism Research Is Shifting Away from Searching for a 'Cure.'"

34. Quoted in Deborah Rudacille, "The Twenty-Something Free Fall," *Spectrum*, March 29, 2017. www.spectrumnews.org.

35. Quoted in "Teens with Autism and Caregivers Should Plan Early for Adulthood," *Science Daily*, January 6, 2016. www.sciencedaily.com.

36. Grandin, *The Autistic Brain*, p. 184.

Chapter 4: How Is Autism Managed?

37. Quoted in Watanabe, "He Couldn't Speak as a Child. Now This Autistic Student is Giving a Commencement Address."

38. Quoted in Watanabe, "He Couldn't Speak as a Child. Now This Autistic Student is Giving a Commencement Address."

39. Quoted in Stenson, "Why the Focus of Autism Research is Shifting Away from Searching for a 'Cure.'"

40. Quoted in Liz Szabo, "Autism Research Unraveling Mysteries," *Arizona Republic*, April 9, 2012. https://archive.azcentral.com.

41. Quoted in Elizabeth DeVita-Raeburn, "The Controversy over Autism's Most Common Therapy," *Spectrum*, August 10, 2016. www.spectrumnews.org.

42. Quoted in Michele C. Hollow, "For Some Children with Autism, Dance Is a Form of Expression," *New York Times*, November 19, 2019. www.nytimes.com.

43. Quoted in Pitney Jr., *The Politics of Autism: Navigating the Contested Spectrum*, p. 12.

44. Quoted in Szabo, "Autism Research Unraveling Mysteries."

45. Quoted in Alisa Opar, "A Medical Condition or Just a Difference? The Question Roils Autism Community," *Washington Post*, May 6, 2019. www.washingtonpost.com.

46. Quoted in Solomon, *Far from the Tree*, p. 282.

For Further Research

Books

Sarah Goldy-Brown, *Autism Spectrum Disorder*. New York: Lucent Press, 2018.

Naoki Higashida, *The Reason I Jump: The Inner Voice of a Thirteen-Year-Old Boy with Autism*. New York: Random House, 2013.

Kris Hirschmann, *Kids and Autism*. San Diego, CA: ReferencePoint Press, 2018.

Sy Montgomery, *Temple Grandin: How the Girl Who Loved Cows Embraced Autism and Changed the World*. New York: Houghton Mifflin, 2012.

Internet Sources

Beth Arky, "Going to College with Autism," *Child Mind Institute*, n.d. https://childmind.org.

"Autism 101," *Spectrum News,* November 5, 2018. www.spectrumnews.org.

Jamie Felzer and Linda Drozdowicz, "Autism, Explained: What Is Autism, and How Can You Identify It?" *ABC News*, April 1, 2019. https://abcnews.go.com.

Temple Grandin, "TED Talk: The World Needs All Kinds of Minds," *TED*, n.d. www.ted.com.

Perri Klass, "The Search for a Biomarker for Early Autism Diagnosis," *New York Times*, April 22, 2019. www.nytimes.com.

Websites

Autistic Self Advocacy Network
https://autisticadvocacy.org

A self-advocacy organization run by and for people on the spectrum, the Autistic Self Advocacy Network promotes autism awareness and advocacy.

CDC: Autism Spectrum Disorder
www.cdc.gov/ncbddd/autism/index.html

The Centers for Disease Control and Prevention's website features a database of information on autism spectrum disorders.

Spectrum News
www.spectrumnews.org

Spectrum News is a comprehensive news site providing news reports and science-based analysis on the latest autism research.

Index

Index Continued

Image Credits

Cover: © pixelheadphoto/iStockphoto
5: © Kathy Hutchins/Shutterstock Images
7: © Photographee.eu/Shutterstock Images
9: © Photographee.eu/Shutterstock Images
12: © Rawpixel.com/Shutterstock Images
15: © Red Line Editorial
19: © SolStock/iStockphoto
23: © Africa Studio/Shutterstock Images
25: © whitehoune/Shutterstock Images
29: © juanestey/iStockphoto
31: © Krakenimages.com/Shutterstock Images
35: © LightHard/Shutterstock Images
36: © T.W. van Urk/Shutterstock Images
43: © Imagesbybarbara/iStockphoto
47: © adamkaz/iStockphoto
48: © Christy Thompson/Shutterstock Images
51: © Manuela Durson/Shutterstock Images
53: © Alena Ozerova/Shutterstock Images
57: © Motortion Films/Shutterstock Images
59: © Photographee.eu/Shutterstock Images
60: © Sergey Novikov/Shutterstock Images
64: © Hailshadow/iStockphoto
66: © SewCream/Shutterstock Images

About the Author

Elisabeth Herschbach is an editor and writer from Washington, DC.